Active Woman's Health Guide

The Active Woman's Health Guide

Dr Wendy Dodds and Paul Wade

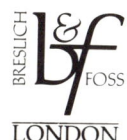

LONDON

Breslich & Foss
Golden House
28-31 Great Pulteney Street
London W1R 3DD
First published 1986

Text © Dr Wendy Dodds and Paul Wade 1986
Photographs, illustrations and design © Breslich & Foss 1986
Concept: Team Wade
Designer: Roger Daniels
Health Editor: Monique Maxwell
Editor: Judy Martin
Photographer: Mike Cowper
Illustrations: Don Parry
Fitness Consultant: Gordon Richards MBE
Additional Research: Katherine Arnold, Monique Maxwell

This book was produced with the help of
Arena UK, a division of Le Coq Sportif

All rights reserved. No part of this
publication may be reproduced in any
form or by any means without permission
of the publishers.

British Library Cataloguing in Publication Data
Dodds, Wendy
 The active woman's health guide.
 1. Women — Health and hygiene
 I. Title II. Wade, Paul
 613'.04244 RA778

ISBN 1 85004 028 1 Hbk
ISBN 1 85004 029 X Pbk

Photoset in Great Britain by Fakenham Photosetting Ltd,
Fakenham, Norfolk
Colour origination by Dot Gradations
Printed by Cambus Litho, East Kilbride, Scotland

Contents

Introduction	7
Why Exercise?	8
Infancy and the Early Years	16
Starting to Exercise	24
Major Body Changes	54
Nutrition and Diet	90
Stress and Addiction	104
Relaxation and Massage	111
Body Care	116
Exercise after Surgery	130
Sport and Exercise Guide	134
Index	156

'Use your health, even to the point of wearing it out. That is what it is for. Spend all you have before you die.'

GEORGE BERNARD SHAW
Preface to *The Doctor's Dilemma*

Introduction

There is increasing evidence that regular exercise is of benefit in promoting a healthy body. In the very young, active games improve neuromuscular co-ordination while in the elderly exercise can maintain mobility and make the activities of daily living easier.

In the past, social pressures may have restricted the range of women's activities, but as it becomes increasingly acceptable for everyone to participate in most sports, it is appreciated that there need be no limitations for women. Indeed, in some activities women may outshine men — horseriding, yachting and long-distance swimming, for example — despite the physiological differences of small heart, smaller lungs, less muscle and more fat. In other areas, such as marathon running, women are rapidly catching up with men. Obviously in the majority of team sports, the disparity in physical strength makes it undesirable for women to compete against men. Just as schoolchildren should ideally be matched for weight and height so, in basic terms should adults.

With the increasing involvement of women in sport, it is important that we should understand our bodies in order to obtain maximum enjoyment from the forms of exercise we choose — and enjoyment is paramount. If exercise is considered a chore, then the physical and mental benefits will be countered. For this reason, it is important to select activities that appeal, to participate in a variety of sports and to try out new ones.

If you are only just beginning to take regular exercise you can let your body adjust gradually to the new routine. Initially there are aches and pains from long-forgotten muscles put into action once again. As you become fitter, these aches will disappear but you must beware of any pain which occurs as you exercise, because this could be a warning that you are overdoing it. You must learn to listen to your body, discovering the pleasures of increasing fitness while watching for the warning signs of stress or injury; and at the same time you can learn to relax yourself, matching your more vigorous activity with the equally regenerating habits of gentle stretching, self-massage and extra sleep.

Regular exercise is fun and there are many rewards from achieving a skilled and successful level in your chosen sport. Whether you like to work out alone, play in a team or join the massed ranks of runners at the start of a marathon, you will benefit from knowing what your body can do, what it needs and how it can be maintained at its best.

Wendy Dodds

Why Exercise?

It has been recognised for thousands of years that exercise, taken little and often, can greatly enhance the quality of life; some even say the duration of life. Although this simple tenet is universally acknowledged today, it is constantly undermined by our largely inactive lifestyles — all in the name of convenience and time-saving. Exercise gives us many things: improved circulation, healthier complexion, increased resistance to infections, diseases, aches and pains; it protects against depression and replaces anxiety with serenity. With exercise, in a word, comes fitness.

Fitness

Fitness is a state of physical—and mental—health which allows us to take part in exercise comfortably and enjoyably so that it doesn't hurt, so that we can look forward to it, laugh, and feel good afterwards. Fitness allows us to get on with our lives at our own natural pace, and to be able to reap its rewards without succumbing to the many stresses which have become inevitable in living in the twentieth century. But the trouble with fitness is that it has been labelled as a fad, putting it into the same category as hula hoops and skate boards: something that will be forgotten after a while.

The pursuit of fitness should be as natural as cleaning your teeth. It needs to be just as regular, and just as thorough: too little effort while cleaning does no good, just as cleaning once a day is too infrequent. And just as some tooth-cleaning addicts will never let a sweet or candy pass their lips, there are exercise junkies who lose sight of the fun and pleasure of sport.

The problem is that, while fitness can only be acquired gradually, there is no easy way to exercise. All the advertisements featuring ladies being pummelled into shape by some sort of machine are rubbish. *There is no substitute for hard work!*

What Are You Exercising?

Quite simply, it's the 40% of the body that consists of muscle. If bones are the hard inner skeleton, then muscles are the softer, more elastic outer skeleton that holds these bones together. They all interconnect and interact, and so it is no use exercising one lot and ignoring the rest.

The Heart

What most people don't realise is that there is one muscle that needs exercise more than any other—the heart—and it is the one muscle that we can never allow to stop working. It has to pump blood round our bodies, enriching it with the oxygen we breathe into our lungs, and then disposing of carbon dioxide and other wastes in the next breath. The blood has to travel through

Women who are Fit

- Cope with stress better
- Are more self-assured
- Have less backache
- Find their skin glows
- Are better prepared for childbirth
- Are less susceptible to hangovers
- Are proud of their bodies
- Awake more refreshed
- Have fewer menstrual problems
- Recover from jetlag sooner
- Don't need to diet
- Usually have easier deliveries
- Have less chance of heart attacks
- Are protected from depression
- Boast a better sex life
- Have healthy-looking hair
- Are less likely to suffer post-natal depression
- Can give up smoking easily
- Are emotionally more stable
- Enjoy life more!

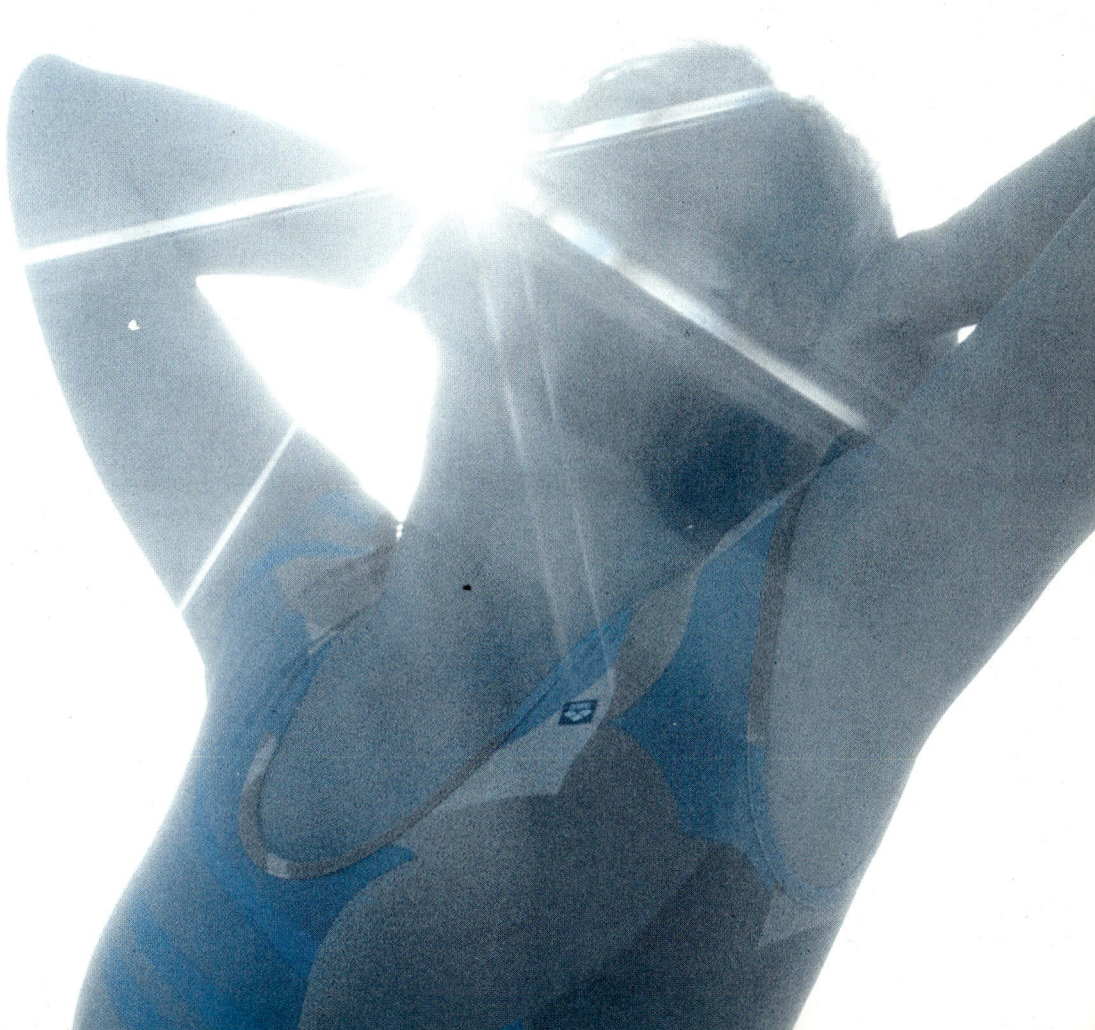

WHY EXERCISE?

many blood vessels, so the more easily it flows the better, and the less work the heart has to do.

However, the Western diet is rich in animal fats, sugars and cholesterol. These substances, when consumed in excess of the body's real needs, have the potential to clog the arteries with fatty deposits (atheroma), rather like limescale in a radiator pipe. The passage through the arteries becomes narrower, and the heart has to pump harder.

The best way to prevent and minimise the blockage (and hence damage to the heart) is to modify your diet and to exercise. It is important to try and combine the two, because each complements the other, and it is easier to stick to a diet/exercise routine. You will also notice the benefits sooner. By working your heart a little harder than usual for at least 10 minutes each day, you will strengthen your heart, enlarge it and enable it to pump more blood, more slowly, with each beat.

Your Heart Rate

Normal Heart Beat	Fit Heart Beat
75 per minute = 100,000 per day	50 per minute = 70,000 per day

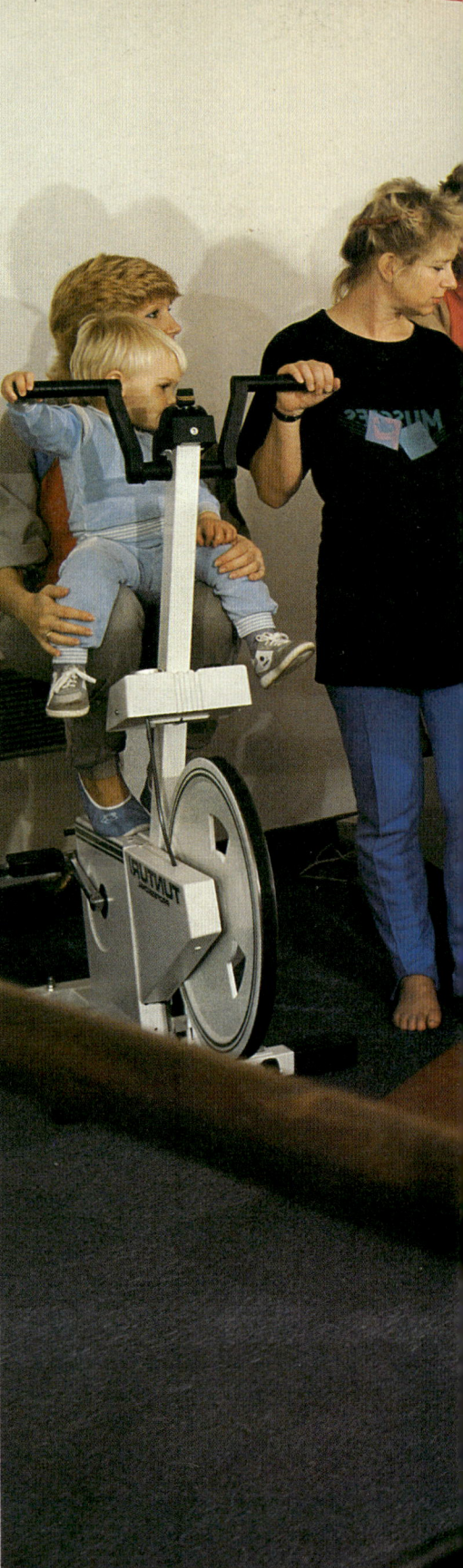

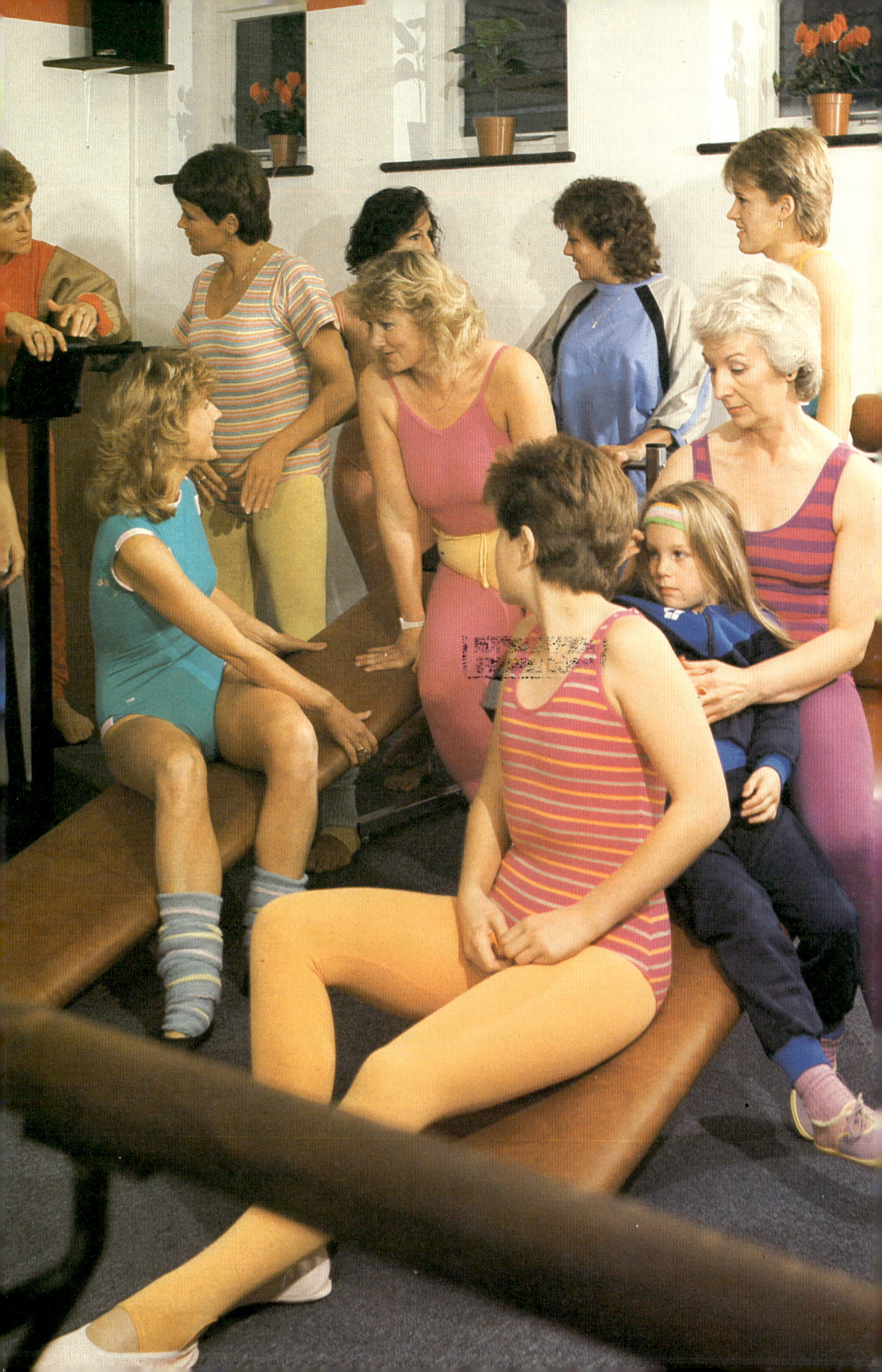

Hard Work

We mentioned hard work, and this means exercising sufficiently vigorously or long enough to raise your pulse rate (ie, heart beat), which in turn means working up a bit of a sweat. Very many people work hard—but at sedentary jobs. However, even the most monotonous of jobs can be fitness-enhancing if you make the most of the opportunities available. In London in 1953, Professor Jeremy Morris analysed the lifestyles of bus drivers and bus conductors. The bus conductors who had to climb up and down the stairs of their double-decker buses selling tickets had less heart attacks and strokes than the drivers who had equally busy days but spent them sitting down. In the USA, twenty years later, Dr Ralph Paffenbarger compared two large groups with different backgrounds. He found that the more active longshoremen (dockers) suffered less heart trouble than the more affluent, but less energetic graduates of Harvard University.

Research into preventative medicine is relatively new because Western doctors have concentrated on finding the cures for cancer and other diseases, and on replacing diseased hearts with new ones. These are wonderful scientific advances, but ones that many experts feel could be countered by encouraging the pursuit of a healthy diet and a healthy and active way of life. While all the studies so far show that exercise has a host of benefits, it is a small Communist country that has proved that prevention is better than cure.

East Germany has a clause in its constitution encouraging 'physical culture and sport as elements of socialist culture (for) the all-round physical and mental development of the citizens'. Furthermore, 'the state ... encourages the participation of citizens in physical culture and sport for the complete expression of the Socialist personality and for the fulfilment of cultural interests and needs'. This has worked so well that East Germany's women have produced outstanding results at international level, and sports medicine expert Dr Kabisch writes that 'simultaneously there has been a shift in emphasis of all medical and social measures, from the mainly curative to the prophylactic'. Doctors can therefore concentrate on the really sick rather than say, the overweight smoker who causes his or her own downfall.

'Something like 6 out of 10 acute hospital admissions are due to the neglect of some health tenet; people are overweight or have high blood pressure. In other words, 6 out of 10 admissions are preventable.' So says Dr Robert Cantu, an American sports medicine expert, emphasising how much and how easily exercise can relieve avoidable illness, stress and strain.

Are You Fit?

Housewives still make up the major proportion of the female population. A woman at home works hard and long, looking after children and husband, cooking meals and washing clothes, running to the shops and cleaning the house. She often holds down an additional job too. Certainly, she is busy, and she may be healthy; but this is not the same as being fit unless some part of the day is spent in working up that sweat-raising pulse. Put simply, you are unfit if you find yourself short of breath when you have to run for a bus, panting when you walk up a flight of stairs, have a daily feeling of tiredness or lethargy, or an inability to get out of bottom gear or through the day without a big effort or the use of stimulants such as caffeine or nicotine.

While the achievements of sportswomen at international level may seem remote from the majority of us, it is these role models who provide us with a wealth of statistics to prove the benefits of exercise as we pass through the complex body changes from new-born to ninety, as we have highlighted in the following chapters.

Women and Sport

The sporting ability of men and women has recently become the subject of comparison, an interesting but unfair and unhelpful exercise. Women *are* different: they menstruate, have babies and feed their young. Psychologically, they also have more staying power and handle stress better. On average, men are stronger and heavier; they have a greater muscle mass. But so what? Mental attitude is more important than physical strength when comparing women with men.

Supporters of Women's Lib' usually concentrate on political and academic freedom, and yet sport is arguably releasing millions of women annually. Mass runs have attracted thousands of women in traditionally conservative countries as far apart as Japan, Brazil and Ireland. Women cricketers in India are watched by tens of thousands, and in 1984 the first Arab woman (and first from the African continent) won an Olympic gold medal when Nawal El Moutawakel (Morocco) took first place in the demanding 400 m hurdles.

Cynics may mock the fanaticism displayed by some women (especially runners), but when this form of liberation is achieved without the benefit of a special education or vast amounts of money it must be applauded, giving as it does, health, friendship and fun for anyone from 0 to 100.

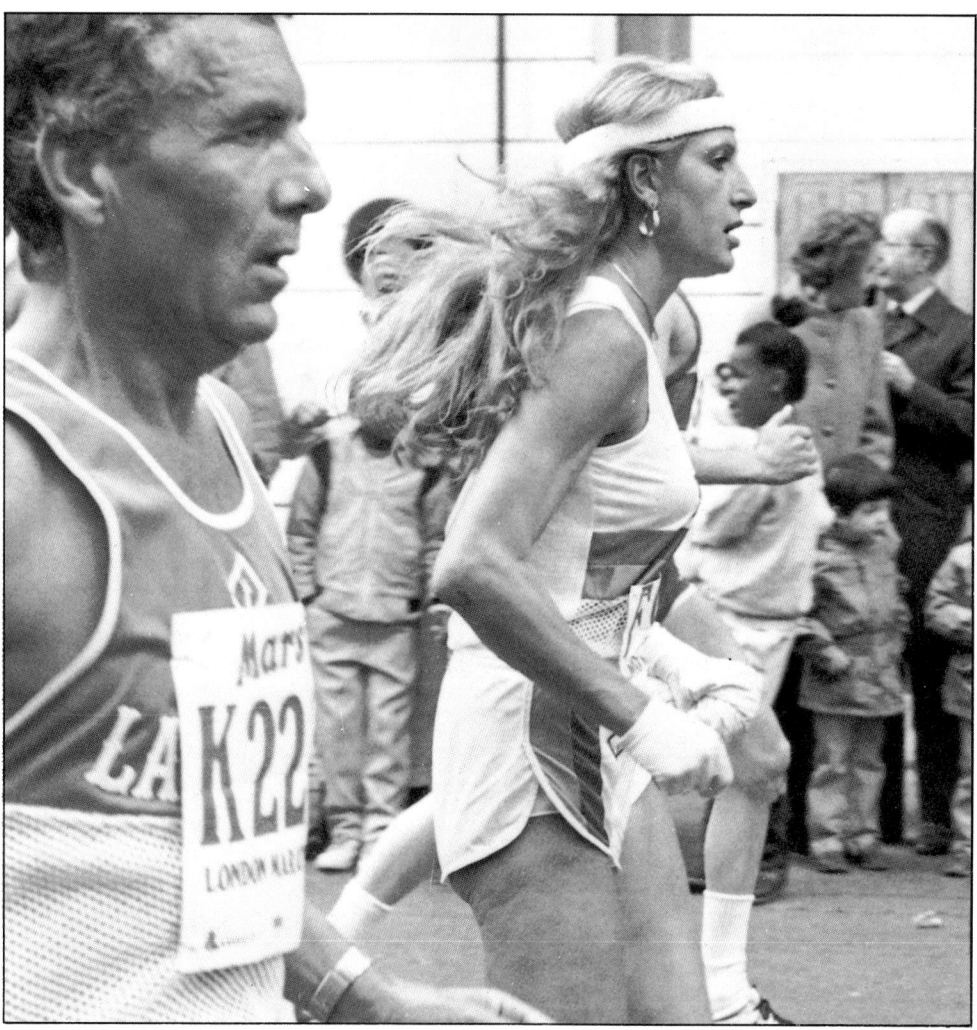

Every year an increasing number of women prove that with regard to physique and stamina, they are at no disadvantage in the arduous test of the marathon, an event until recently considered an exclusively male preserve.

WHY EXERCISE?

Exercise and the Disabled

In many ways, the disabled show able-bodied women the way when it comes to recognising the benefits of exercise and sport. After the Second World War, Professor Ludwig Guttman set up the now famous sports programme at Stoke Mandeville Hospital, England, to rehabilitate disabled men and women. The effects—both physical and mental—are now recognised worldwide, and here, a group of sportswomen at the British Disabled Waterski Association explain why sport and exercise are such an important part of their lives.

Freda Horrocks has been blind since birth. She went to a special school where she had to learn to swim. 'It took a lot of persuasion because I was terrified at first. If I had been at home with my parents I'm sure they would have let me off to be kind to me. But parents can be too soft, so I'm glad the teachers persisted because swimming was a breakthrough for me.' Freda has run the London Marathon and waterskis, too!

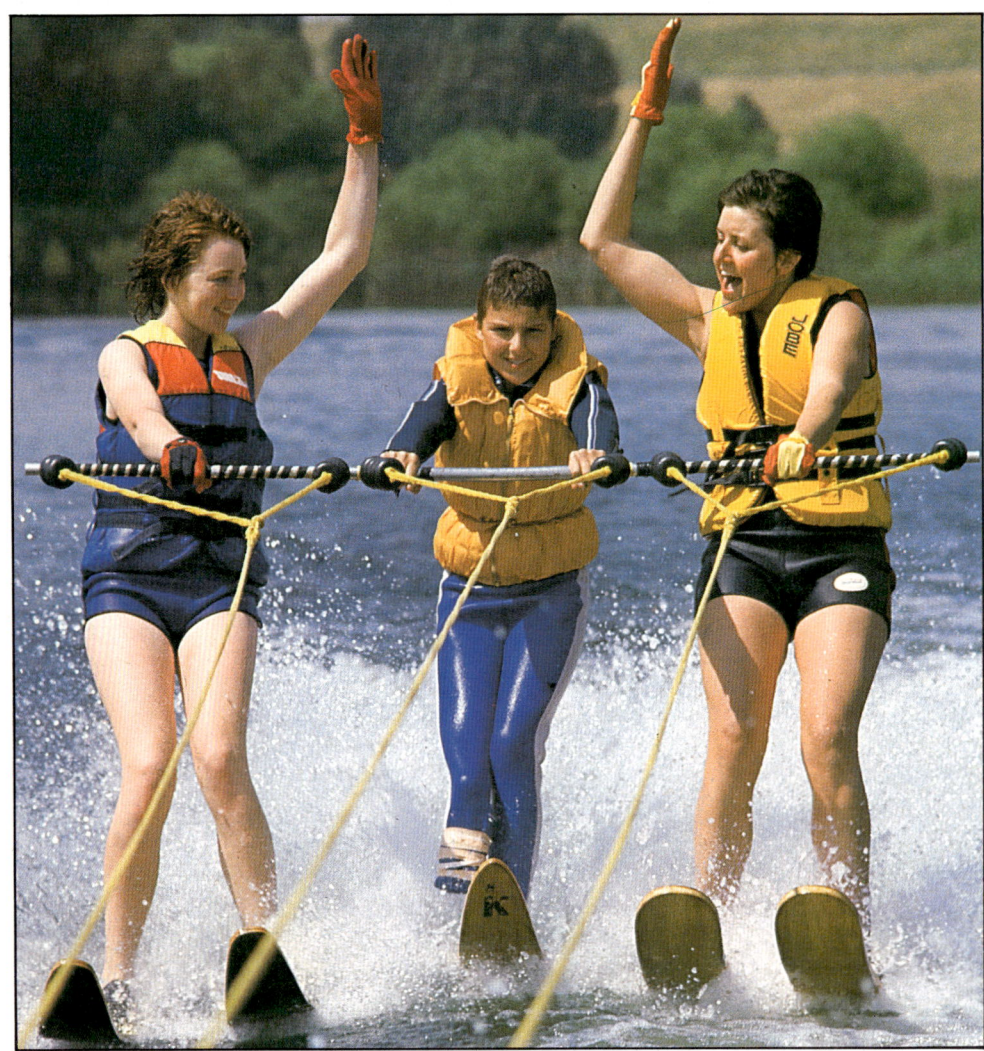

Julie Hunt aged 12, waterskiing on Heron lake barely six months after a miracle operation for cancer of the thigh. Intrepid Julie has also learnt to ice skate and parascend.

Jayne Harrison, now 21, is also partially sighted. She remembers when she was 12. 'I didn't want to be different from my friends and found that swimming improved my muscle co-ordination and strength and gave me extra confidence.' Now she waterskis even though she feels she has no natural sense of balance. 'That's not because of lack of sight, that's just me.'

Debbie Simms, now 18, had 40 operations after bone cancer was diagnosed at 13. She lost part of a lung and her leg, above the knee: 'At first I just wanted to sit around but my Mum made me wear the artificial leg even though I kept falling over. I didn't fancy swimming because I felt everyone would be looking at me.' But she got over that self-consciousness and joined in with the rest of the kids at school: 'The teacher would say, "We're doing high jump and long jump; what are you doing?" and I'd say, "High jump and long jump, same as you".' Now Debbie is a gold medallist in waterski slalom at the Disabled Olympics and feels 'nothing is impossible. There's always something you can do even if a bit of you is missing'. In fact, if she didn't exercise she'd have trouble breathing and moving with only one lung and one leg.

Viv Orchard, 19, was school games captain and very active when she slipped and fell and was run over by a train at 18. 'My periods stopped for a while afterwards due to the drugs and the shock. Once you've left school it takes more determination to stay fit.' She waterskis and does aerobics once a week even though she says in all honesty 'I do it for the result, not for the pure enjoyment of the sport.' She goes to discos with her friends and 'if I fall over because my artificial leg slips, I just get up and keep on dancing'.

Janice Newman, 40, is registered blind. 'My sight seemed to go overnight when I was 7 though I could still distinguish bright objects. So I enjoyed playing field hockey where I could see the white ball against the ground; giving it a good whack got rid of my frustration and aggression'. In her mid-20s she did a lot of long-distance walking and hill climbing but does less now as her sight has deteriorated further. But she still runs and goes cross-country skiing. 'I take pride in my body. I like to keep it supple, slim and strong.' She now is learning tricks on skis—going backwards is the next step! 'You have to get over your doubt in your own ability. That takes determination but the exhilaration of success is worth it.'

The most extreme and heartening success for a disabled woman came in 1982 at the 12th Commonwealth Games in Brisbane, Australia when 38-year-old archer Neroli Fairhall of New Zealand won the gold medal. She was the first paraplegic to win a major title in open competition. Confined to a wheelchair since losing the use of her legs in a motorcycle accident in 1969, she was asked afterwards if she had an advantage in shooting from a seated position. 'I can't answer that,' she replied, 'I've never shot an arrow standing up.'

Exercise for the mentally handicapped is also a boon. John F Kennedy's sister, Eunice Kennedy Shriver, set up *'Let's Play to Grow'*, a world-wide campaign to encourage activity among handicapped children. It has been so successful that many are now joining in able-bodied activities, including gymnastics, with confidence. A permanent Sports Club has been set up at the Monyhull Hospital in Birmingham, England which concentrates on the 17–35 year olds who suffer more from mental than physical handicaps. As they have grown up in fairly confined areas with few sports areas or facilities (let alone little encouragement) they have poor physical fitness, are often overweight and lack basic hand-eye co-ordination. This in turn makes them unco-ordinated and clumsy in everyday life which depresses their confidence. The Sports Club reverses these trends quite dramatically with a programme mapped out by remedial gymnast Alison Dines which seeks to improve co-ordination and balance, strength and stamina, posture and intellectual development, as well as encouraging teamwork, socialisation and integration. What is more, it boosts morale and is fun!

Infancy and the Early Years

Just as the years from infancy to early school are important in terms of mental development, a child's physical ability is growing and developing at the same time. Training your child to habits of exercise can be fun — not a chore — for both of you and from the earliest months there are steps you can take to encourage strong and healthy development.

Birth to Two Years

The first two years of a girl's life involve the fastest growth period. Growth is irregular, coming in spurts which are governed by external factors like the season of the year (slow in the autumn, faster in the spring), nutrition, and internal factors like bones, muscles and fat. These all grow at different rates.

The Head

Most noticeable is the size of a baby's head, which is about a quarter of the size of the body at birth—reflecting the complex developments that occur in the early years. In fact the circumference of the head grows by about 25% in the first year and a mere 15% in the next eleven years!

The Body

If the brain is the fastest developing part of the body, then the protection against infection provided by the lymph glands comes second, followed by the bones. Basically, a baby grows and develops from the top downwards.

Reflexes

New-born babies may look hopeless and helpless, but they are born with some important reflexes, although these disappear a few weeks after birth. These reflexes are used by doctors to check that the baby's brain is functioning normally.

0–1 Month: Supported, a baby looks as if she knows how to walk, with a curious 'stepping' action.

0–3 Months: Offered a finger, a baby grips it tightly. You can even pull her up by her grip.

0–8 Months: A baby can swim under water *instinctively*, eyes open, fearless and holding her breath.

With this in mind, Professor Lieselote Diem carried out considerable research in West Germany encouraging babies as small as two months to float on their backs and fronts and even, by five months, to propel themselves through the water before they had learned to walk! The Cologne-based professor also

INFANCY AND THE EARLY YEARS

encouraged dry land activity in babies, and discovered that in later years they had more energy and drive, had better leadership skills and were more adaptable to change. Her other finding—that early swimmers seemed brighter—has been backed by studies in Czechoslovakia where Dr Koch found that 'water babies' knew twice as many words as non-swimmers by the age of twenty months. In West Germany, researchers at Munich University measured the physical development of tiny swimmers and found that they quickly increased their lung capacity by about 20% and that this simultaneously aided brain development because of the extra oxygen in the blood.

The reason researchers have used swimming for their enquiry is that the gentle resistance provided by water helps develop the heart, lungs and muscles. They even argue that the reduction in the effect of gravity can speed up the messages sent back to the brain by the nervous system. However, swimming aside, there can be no doubt that involving young children in new sensations and encouraging them to explore new horizons is startlingly beneficial.

The value of parents helping their baby learn to swim is psychologically important too. The child is being taught to do something enjoyable by the parent, trusts the parent and learns elementary discipline. And if that isn't enough, Professor Diem maintains that these swimmers sleep and eat better and develop better concentration. What is more, as the muscles develop, posture improves. Some doctors worry that swimming before six months leaves a baby open to infection, but again all the studies seem to prove the reverse—that children develop greater resistance.

Mother and baby classes are growing in popularity in sport and leisure centres and clubs. In her book, *Swim, Baby, Swim*, Anne Hawley spells out the fun to be had by the mother and child exercising in this way.

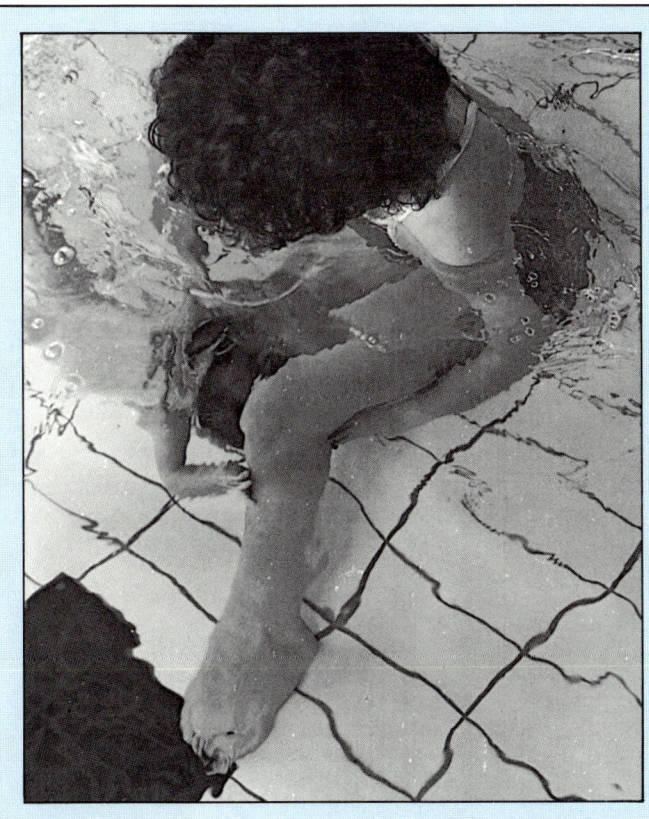

❛ Instinctively, a baby controls its breathing when placed under water and very young babies haven't learnt to fear water: now is the time to encourage and develop these natural instincts. ... It is obvious from my classes that babies who learn to develop their swimming abilities at an early stage are normally very alert and astute for their age. They also progress much more quickly in their crawling and walking abilities. Swimming sessions for baby are undoubtedly the best exercise she can take before the age of two years. Most babies spend their first six months just eating and sleeping, but 'swim babies' eat, sleep and exercise. ❜

SWIM, BABY, SWIM

Co-ordination

Every childcare book has average times for how long it takes a baby to develop into a co-ordinated, active child. The figures can only be *average*, and on a planet supporting 3 billion human beings there are millions who are quicker and millions who are slower to reach various stages of development. So never panic if your child fails to meet the average. This is quite normal, and in the end they all catch up. Even children who suffer a debilitating weakness early on in life will eventually catch up, given the help and encouragement all youngsters need.

As a child develops her temporary reflexes are lost and gradually replaced with more purposeful movements (see chart, below). While this is drawn up as a month by month guide, it is the *order* rather than the timing of each development which you might find a useful guide.

Feet

Babies should be encouraged to go bare foot as often as possible. This helps to develop balance through a greater awareness of the toes and the flexibility of the foot. It is worth remembering, too, that tight socks can be just as restricting as tight shoes at this formative stage.

Left or Right Handed?

By about eighteen months, children seem to work out whether they are naturally left- or right-handed. About 10% of the world's population is left-handed, and most people now realise that attempts to force children away from their left-handedness can actually cause psychological problems. For girls, the percentage is just below 10% but there are real advantages in sporting terms. In fact an abnormal number of star players in some sports (ie, tennis, 20%, and also fencing) are 'lefties'.

Major Stages of Development

MONTHS	SITTING	HOLDING	STANDING
4	Can hold head up in line with body	Can hold light object (eg plastic ring) when put in hands	Stepping reflex forgotten
5	Can lift head forward to 'help'	Can pick up an object—usually two handed	Kicking and playing with toes
6	Neck and back muscles develop and the idea of sitting is easier to cope with	Picks up object with whole hand; does not appreciate use of fingers as separate entities	'Baby Bouncer' can be introduced. Ensure correct height off ground with toes just touching. Use in 30–45 minute sessions
7	Babies can sit up for a few seconds	Can feed herself holding a biscuit. Can switch objects from hand to hand	Starts to pull up on furniture to move around room
8–9	Can lean forward, turn and look for objects at side or behind	Enjoys dropping and handing you objects—though not quite sure *how* you let go! Also uses several fingers and thumb	Walking frame can be fun—but use in short bursts to avoid over-reliance
10–12	Confident and in control	Now uses one finger and thumb for largish objects. Plays pat-a-cake and waves	Can walk with support. Gradually learns to walk unaided—although this can take until 18 months

INFANCY AND THE EARLY YEARS

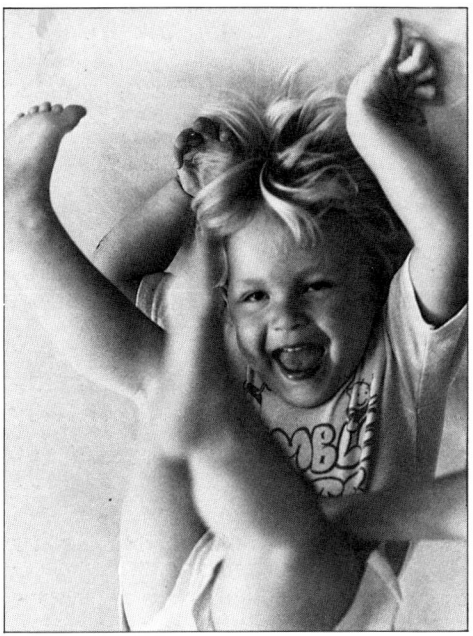

Exercise and Play

Just as teachers have developed watersport as a fun way to introduce children to exercise, so new and interesting ways of encouraging children's play are being used on dry land. One example is *Tumble Tots* developed by two British Olympic gymnastics coaches, Bill Cosgrave and Nik Stuart. They recognised that children growing up in urban society are deprived of the freedom to develop balance, agility, co-ordination etc. Since playgrounds cater for bigger kids and parents worry about roads, young children rarely have access to fields or other places where they can climb, swing and jump safely on spring turf. A child living in a small house that is not 'child-proof', with valuable china or dangerous pan handles or fireplaces is often left in a play-pen. Useful for a few minutes at a time, play-pens can also cause frustration, even retard development. *Tumble Tots* goes the other way, positively encouraging a child's natural acrobatic ability.

Nik Stuart and Bill Cosgrave have quantified the sort of development they have seen amongst youngsters who have participated in their *Tumble Tots* scheme. They insist that this is play, but play with a purpose. Despite the expertise, it is not an elitist programme to produce champion gymnasts. Nor is it for those parents keen to inflate their own egos by some reflected glory from offspring 'out-tumbling' the others. Each child is different, each develops both physically and socially to the beat of their own drum.

What Parents Can Do

More primary motor skills (ways of making the body do what you want) are learned in the first two years than at any other time in your life. This is why parental help and stimulation are so important. Some experts think that *all* primary motor skills are learned by the age of four, and that any skills thereafter are variations on a theme. So, while parents may not want a 'clumsy' child they may be unwilling to help the child to be 'athletic' in the simplest sense. But help, in the form of simple games, maintaining the fun element all the time (*never* introducing competition) will help a child to enjoy this form of learning as well as other forms of education like talking, learning new words and reading.

While swimming or *Tumble Tots* are wonderful ideas, they are not available to everyone, and need expert supervision, too. But there are plenty of other simple games worth trying:

- Roll a ball (medium size) towards your baby to stimulate the idea of judging distance and following a moving object, as well as stopping or trapping it.
- Encourage the idea of kicking a ball—using *both* feet, starting with ball stationary.
- In a safe space, encourage your youngster to throw a small ball. It will go in every direction but the right one, but helps develop awareness of 'above me', 'behind me', etc. Encourage the use of both hands.
- As soon as your child uses a wooden spoon or stick to hit things, develop hand–eye co-ordination by hitting:
  a) a stationary ball,
  b) a ball rolled towards her,
  c) a bouncing ball.
  Again, use of both hands is encouraged.

19

INFANCY AND THE EARLY YEARS

Two to Six Years: certain physical abilities you can expect

2 YEAR OLD

- Jumps down and lands on two feet without the use of her hands (from waist height at least)
- Does forward roll in a straight path, by understanding how to tuck in her head, and being able to use hands for balance during the roll
- Understands different shapes—ie, lines, curves, angles
- Able to catch a ball in the air at head height. Also to roll a ball towards and away
- Pushes or kicks a ball with foot in a predetermined path
- Walks properly, runs, and runs and jumps to land on both feet simultaneously
- Climbs stairs, but one level at a time, so both feet are together.

3 YEAR OLD

- Executes a forward roll and finishes roll tidily in a rounded, tucked position
- Remembers basic sequential order
- Basic ball skills: catching with two hands at various distances; controlling a moving ball with the feet or hands
- Develops a respect for other children, co-operation within a group, and awareness of surroundings
- Rides tricycle
- Climbs stairs properly.
- Jumping from a shoulder height distance, lands on two feet without using hands

4 YEAR OLD

- Ball skills: dribbling while moving; catching ball at various levels; controls and traps moving ball with the hands and feet; kicks and throws ball at a near target
- Grasps position and placement of hands for backward roll
- Can run fast, swerve and turn easily, hop, skip and jump
- Catching is still difficult.
- Runs, walks, skips, jumps and controls momentum safely
- Rolls in a tuck position
- Stands on one foot (Stork stand)

5 YEAR OLD

- *Danger*: legs are strong now so kids can climb and swim unaided—*watch out*!
- Can ride a tricycle fast—or even a 2-wheel bike!
- Can swing, slide and skip alone.

6 YEAR OLD

- Between $5\frac{1}{2}$ and 7 years there is usually a growth spurt and scientists find that exercise (in reasonable amounts) encourages muscles, tendons and bones to grow.
- Catching still a problem: judging path/flight of ball in air
- The most active age yet
- Likes to show off expertise

Two to Six Years

Although the first two years are important, parents should not think that their efforts to play with, and encourage their children, should start to decrease. From two to six, children develop their skills and learn new ones —such as riding a tricycle or skipping. But as the youngsters get more mobile they are more exhausting and demanding which can exasperate parents who expected life to get easier! Meanwhile, growth has slowed down dramatically: the average weight increase in a child's third year is 5 lbs (2·25 kg)—compared to 7 lbs (3·15 kg) in the second year—and maintains a gentle annual drop thereafter.

Seven Years

By now all the motor controls work, so further physical development tends to be based on strength. Also about now, boys and girls seem to separate into their own groups although much of this could be put down to 'sexual stereotyping' by parents, school systems and other organisations. Mothers may well—even subconsciously—encourage their daughters to 'settle down', to follow traditional feminine pursuits. This is about the worst thing you can do.

A Base for Life

Experts agree that seven is the age when the 'building blocks' for complicated skills of sport really work together. Up until now, children will have learnt all the basics but at seven, the demands of sport (accuracy, consistency, etc) are cemented into a person—like the never-forgotten skill of riding a bicycle.

Girls should continue to enjoy the same sports as boys. Quite often they are the same size as boys and even outgrow them in the next couple of years as they approach puberty. If girls stop doing sport and exercise, it will count against them later in life. How many women, enthused by the recent surge of interest in health and exercise have tried to take up a sport and found it impossible to hit a ball or catch it? Meanwhile their equally out-of-shape male partner seems to slip into some sort of groove . . .

It really does seem astonishing that a man's experience as a boy seems to stay with him and that women who were deprived of that extra development,

What do the Doctors Think?

In the USA, the Committee on the Paediatric Aspects of Physical Fitness, Recreation and Sports offered guidelines regarding participation in sports by girls and young women':

- Postpubescent girls should not participate against boys in heavy collision sports because of the grave risk of serious injury due to their lesser muscle mass per unit of body weight.

- The talented female athlete should only participate on a team with boys in an appropriate sport and provided that the school or community offers opportunities for all girls to participate in comparable activities.

- Girls can compete against boys in any sports activity if matched for size, weight, skill and physical maturation.

- Girls can attain high levels of physical fitness through strenuous conditioning activities to improve their physical fitness, agility, strength, appearance, endurance, and sense of physical well-being. These have no unfavourable influence on menstruation, future pregnancy, or childbirth.

- There is no reason to separate prepubescent children by sex in sports, physical education, and recreational activities.

that cementing of the blocks, miss out. However, this does not mean that girls should suddenly be pushed into softball, tennis or hockey. Some sports require a complex combination of skills, all developed to a high level before competence is achieved. Most sports have their own building block schemes like 'short tennis' (played with smaller rackets) or 'mini basketball' (played with lower baskets).

The best interests of girls and women in sports activities are served by opportunities to experience the thrill of sports competition when they are able to qualify for girls' programmes sponsored just for them. Ultimate benefits are greater when efforts are directed to developing girls' programmes and the athletes within them, rather than emphasising the exceptional female athlete who may wish to participate with boys on their terms. What's more, studies show that when it comes to injuries at play, these are reduced by taking part in organised games rather than leaving girls to 'mess around' on their own in playgrounds.

The benefits of organised games are not purely sporting: learning rules is educational, quick thinking becomes mandatory, and the idea of helping and encouraging team-mates is fostered.

Running: Some of the 'old' games are the best. The fun of a three-legged race or a sack race is as great now as it has always been. Careful observation by parents or organisers can build in handicaps so that the fastest and slowest are paired and so on.

Obstacle races are always fun as kids love to crawl and climb. Make up your own course using available materials.

Throwing: Piggy-in-the-middle helps to develop catching, jumping and mobility and is a forerunner of sports like basketball and netball. Throwing a ball for distance or accuracy is also useful in several sports later in life.

Jumping: Sports scientists use a jumping test to find out how much natural spring is in our legs. The same test can be carried out just for fun by kids. Take a piece of chalk and get them to mark a wall as high as possible.

The Right Encouragement

In many Western countries, sport at school has become the victim of budgetary cuts. As a result, many parents (especially if they can afford the time and money) take on the role of sports organisers, coaches and trainers, often with tremendous enthusiasm. On the surface, this seems laudable. But there are question marks about the validity of entrusting children to unskilled but keen amateurs. Some sports like Little League Baseball make you fit, but the extra specific training needed should be guided by an expert. Other sports like soccer can be overly competitive, concentrating on tactics, matches and winning, rather than skill development, fun and participation. How often has a parent acted out his or her frustrated athletic career on the sidelines through a willing offspring? Parents should work *with* experts, helping and encouraging, but not taking over, unless they are prepared to take courses that give them the qualifications to look after children.

As Dorothy Einon points out in her book *Creative Play*:

> There is nothing ... wrong with children taking part in sport, as long as they do so in their own way ... In children's games, children's rules apply; the game can stop while laces are tied or someone gains their breath, and no one bothers too much with the score. But in the mini-leagues, the ethos changes: the child cannot say 'I wasn't ready' and expect another go ... Winning is important and will be remembered beyond the game.

The reason for encouraging sport at this age is not to produce a Wimbledon winner, an Olympic gold medallist or a golfing superstar, but rather to get used to the idea that regular exercise is *fun* —not only in childhood but also on into adulthood and through into old age. That is why variety is to be encouraged, even if special talent seems to be apparent at an early age. And if team games and other organised sports have little appeal, search around in the exercise-related disciplines of dance and movement. Lead by example.

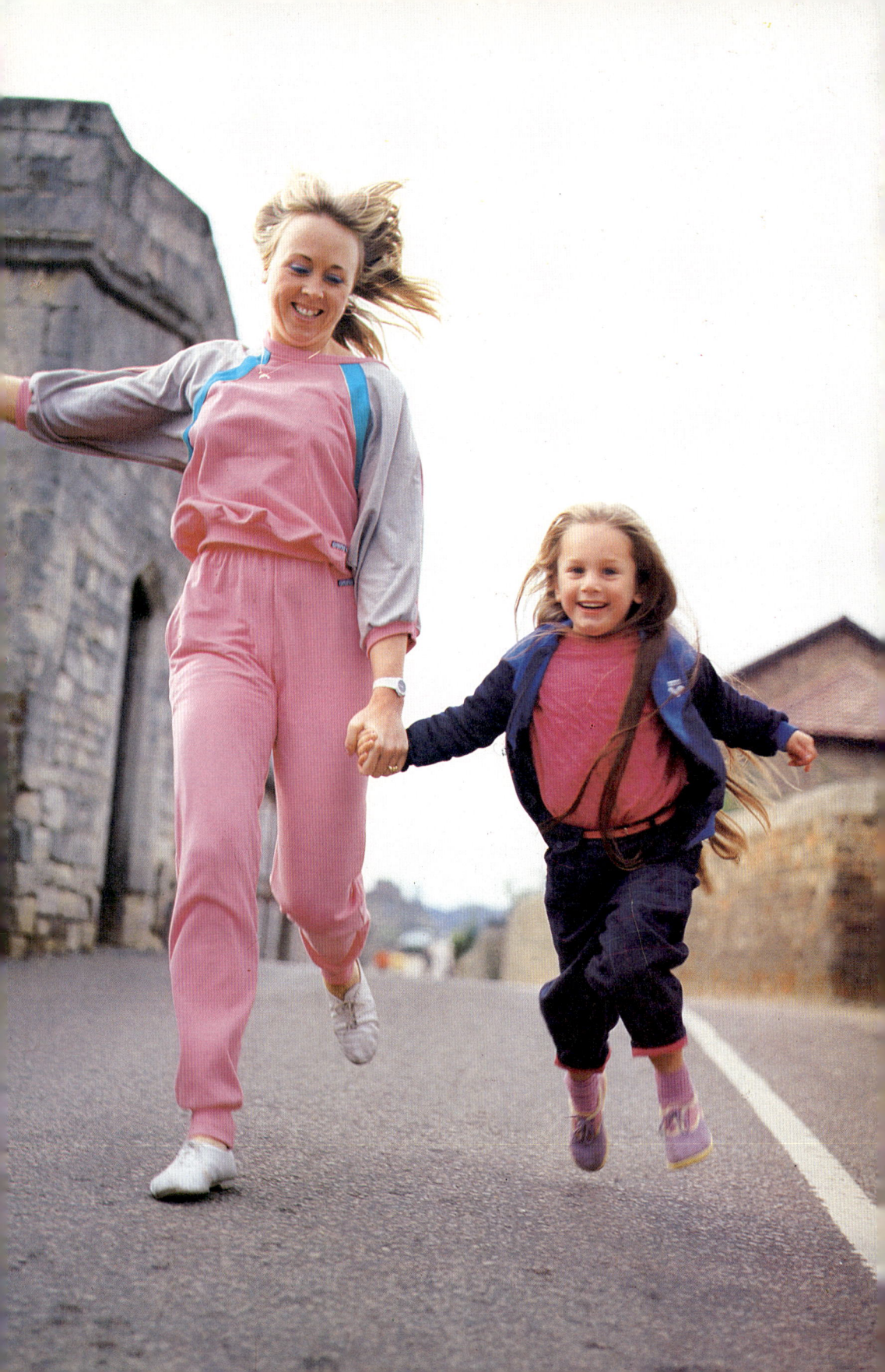

Starting to Exercise

The theory that exercise does you good has been proven time and time again. The problem of taking up exercise, however — especially after a long period of inactivity — has never really been solved. This is probably because there is no easy way of going about it. Exercise, like everything else worth having in life, requires hard work and discipline. But the benefits are quickly felt, giving added impetus to your will to continue.

How Fit Are You?

As we outlined in Chapter One, fitness will benefit your heart first and foremost. The fitter you are, the slower —and more efficient—will be your heart beat, and the better your body will function. Someone who is unfit only uses a quarter of the energy obtained from food, whereas a fit person uses nearly two-thirds—which is why you don't need extra food when you exercise.

The quickest way to tell if you're getting fit is to monitor your heart beat. Take your pulse every day, note down the number of beats per minute and compare pulse rates over a period of time—say, a month. Usually, the pulse is detected by feeling for the artery on the inside of the wrist, although in some people this is not easy to find. There is a much stronger pulse (carotid artery) in your neck: about 2 inches (5 cm) below your ear on the side of your throat. Use a watch (a digital or sweep second hand) to count the beats for fifteen seconds, then multiply the answer by four to give you the number of beats per minute.

Your Ideal Weight

Another feature of getting fit is being the right weight for your height and build. The problem is that most height for weight charts are devised by consulting life insurance companies who only produce statistics to cover the average person. Their results are therefore based on what everyone's size *is* rather than what it should be. Subsequently, many charts give women a false impression of what weight is regarded as a 'fit' weight. What is more, body weight is also governed by build or frame. The thickness of wrists and ankles, usually the least fleshy parts of the body, provides an indicator of whether you have a light or heavy frame. Take this into account when setting yourself a target fitness weight.

You might find that as you get fitter you weigh *more*. This is because you are converting fat into muscle—heavier than fat—which is a good sign. But if your skin is firm, your waist well-defined, and there is an obvious gap at the top of your legs between your thighs, then you are not overweight.

STARTING TO EXERCISE

Simple Heart Test

- Take your pulse first thing on awakening while still in bed, or after you have been lying down and relaxing for about five minutes.
- Get up slowly and stand for about 10–15 seconds before taking your pulse again.
- Note the difference between your pulse rates when lying down and standing up. For example, if your lying down pulse is 50 beats per minute, and your standing up pulse 55 beats per minute, then the difference is 5.
- Compare your result with the chart to see how fit or unfit you are.
- Record your pulse rates in a notebook and see how you improve once you start our exercise plans. Even if you work-out gently, you should see an improvement within a week. If there is no drop in the difference within a month, then you are not working out hard enough.

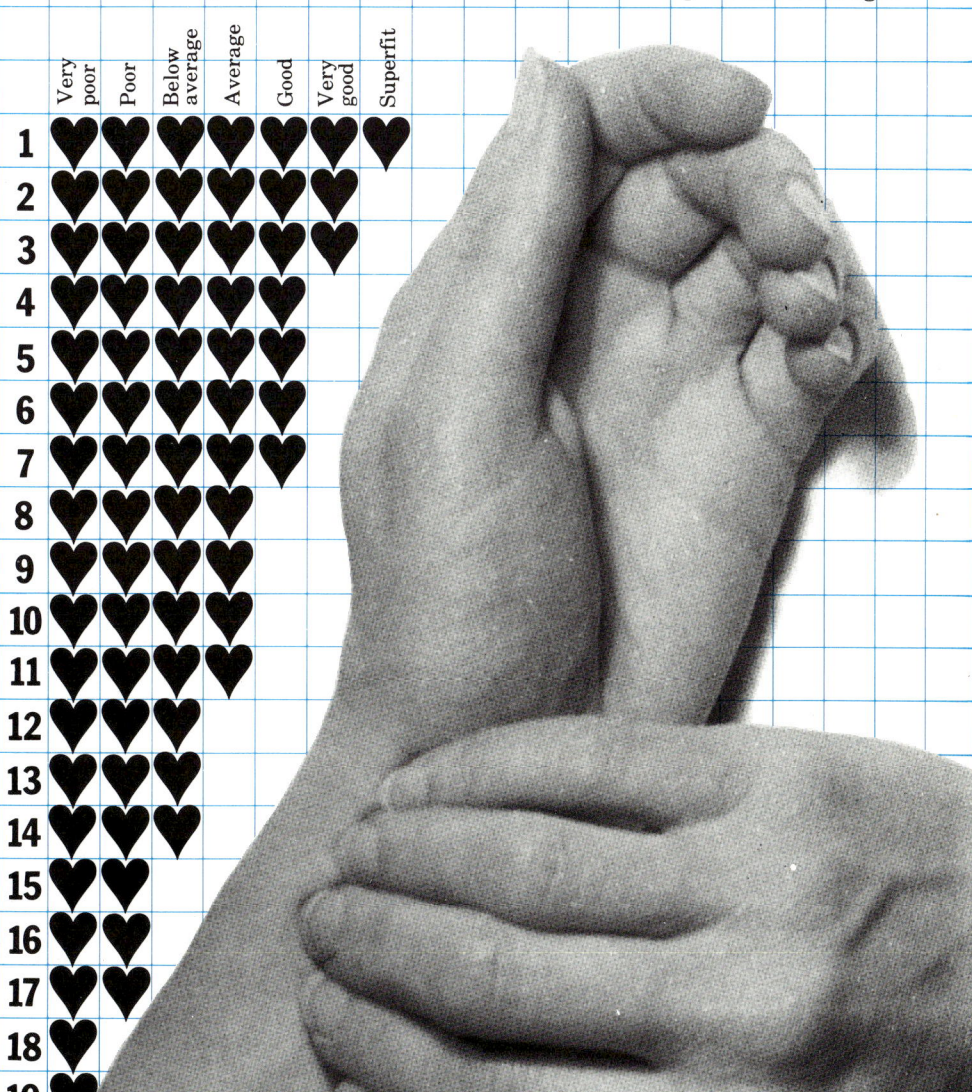

Difference in beats per minute	Very poor	Poor	Below average	Average	Good	Very good	Superfit
1	♥	♥	♥	♥	♥	♥	♥
2	♥	♥	♥	♥	♥	♥	
3	♥	♥	♥	♥	♥		
4	♥	♥	♥	♥			
5	♥	♥	♥	♥			
6	♥	♥	♥	♥			
7	♥	♥	♥	♥			
8	♥	♥	♥				
9	♥	♥	♥				
10	♥	♥	♥				
11	♥	♥	♥				
12	♥	♥					
13	♥	♥					
14	♥	♥					
15	♥	♥					
16	♥	♥					
17	♥	♥					
18	♥						
19	♥						

Exercise is for Everyone

Overweight
Strictly speaking, you should lose weight *in order to get fit* and take up sport or exercise, and not take up exercise to lose weight. This is particularly the case if you are more than 14 lbs (6·5 kg) heavier than your ideal weight (see p. 28). The heavier you are, the greater the strain on your heart, joints and ligaments—and when you start exercising your hips, knees and ankles will take a real pounding. Combining exercise with sound dietary measures (see p. 90) is the most sensible and effective way to lose weight provided you 'break your body in' gradually, observe these recommendations and don't opt for a short, sharp shock treatment.

Over 40
Age is not (and never should be) a bar to taking up exercise or sport (see p. 87). But use your commonsense: don't take up downhill skiing with a slightly arthritic hip! Even as early as 35 years, certain ageing processes are taking place: increase in body fat, decrease in heart performance, oxygen uptake, strength and flexibility. But you can forestall this process by as much as ten years if you take up exercise, although initially you will have to be more patient. Don't rush at getting fit or expect miracle results overnight. Changes will occur—almost immediately—but may not be perceived by you for a couple of weeks.

Smokers
If you smoke, you *can* exercise and you *should* exercise to improve your body's utilisation of oxygen. Ideally, you should stop smoking before you begin our fitness programme to prepare your ailing heart and lungs for the extra oxygen they'll have to cope with, but if you can't face giving up then start The Basic Exercise Plan programme anyway. You'll soon find that you don't want to smoke as much and later, not at all! Surprisingly enough, smokers can achieve quite a high oxygen uptake through regular exercise. Although it will probably seem like very hard work at first, you'll surprise yourself, but you'll never quite be able to catch up with non-smokers.

High Blood Pressure
This is a serious condition requiring regular medical surveillance and, perhaps, medication. One of the long-term benefits of regular exercise is more efficient heart performance and a low but healthy blood pressure. While aiming for this in the long term is laudable, it would be foolish (and dangerous) to undertake vigorous exercise with simply this end in mind. Talk to your doctor: tell him you want to take up an exercise programme, show him this book and ask if there are any extra precautions you should take. If you do experience dizzy spells, headache, or sudden pain during your workout, don't stop suddenly, but slow right down, walk and keep moving—don't slump into a chair!

Heart Disease
If you have any form of heart disease, it is inadvisable to take up any form of exercise (except walking) without first consulting your doctor or cardiologist.

Epilepsy
If you are well-controlled on anticonvulsants, there is no reason why you should not exercise. Be wary of certain 'triggering' factors— eg, going for a long run or workout and then not eating the rest of the day. Also, avoid contact sports and loud, crowded, reverberating swimming pools, and never swim alone.

Diabetes

If you're diabetic and well-controlled on insulin, oral hypoglycaemic drugs, diet, or a combination of these, you can exercise. You will however, have to adjust your insulin, medication and diet accordingly, so talk to your doctor about how to go about it. When you start our fitness programme, remember to take extra special care of your feet and make sure you wear the proper shoes. Diabetics are more prone to infection, and may have impaired circulation and reduced sensation in the feet.

Arthritis

This general term refers to the many types of inflammation or disease of joints. If arthritis affects the lower limbs then it is better to take non-weight bearing exercises such as swimming, cycling or even horse-riding. The limiting factor to the exercise will be pain and this should influence the type and amount of exercise that is taken.

Asthma

This narrowing of the breathing passages—resulting in shortness of breath—may result from an allergy but in older subjects it is commonly a spontaneous occurrence. In some people it may be triggered by exercise. However, swimming is usually well-tolerated as the warm, moist air reduces the chance of an asthmatic attack. With the introduction of drugs and inhalers for asthma most sports can be enjoyed and there are many outstanding sports women who perform at the top level internationally despite regular treatment for asthma.

Low Back Pain

There are many causes of this very common complaint. Frequently, mechanical factors produce abnormal stresses and strains on the ligaments and other supporting structures of the spine. They can be minimised by taking care with bending, lifting and posture. Low back pain in itself should not prevent exercise being taken although certain activities such as road running may make the pain worse. Symptoms may be prevented by avoiding obesity and maintaining good abdominal muscle tone.

Occasionally the pain is severe, spreading into the legs as a result of disturbed mechanical factors in the spine. This causes increased pressure on one of the nerves emerging from the spine which is often referred to as a slipped or prolapsed disc. If this happens, it is necessary to have complete bed rest. Sporting activity except swimming should be avoided. As the pain subsides activity can gradually be resumed.

Depression

Although it is difficult to motivate yourself to exercise when depressed, there is increasing evidence that aerobic exercise can protect against and relieve depression. In people who are already depressed, aerobic exercise sustained for at least 30 minutes five times a week, can have a remarkable anti-depressant effect. The reasons for this are not clear, but are probably mediated by biochemical actions and the release of natural 'pleasure-inducing' chemicals (endorphins). There is also the positive action and willpower needed to get out of the door and the sense of achievement afterwards which can do much to increase self-esteem and motivate self-determination.

Pregnancy

See p. 67.

After Surgery

See p. 130.

STARTING TO EXERCISE

Your Physical Potential

Body Shape
You only have to look at women on the beach to realise that we are all shapes and sizes. Experts have studied this phenomenon for some time and can not only categorise us but also advise us on the best sport and exercise for our particular build. The three basic outlines are ectomorph, mesomorph and endomorph, technical names for tall and skinny, medium and 'just right', and short and broad. These can be subdivided again into a total of six groups.

Muscle Fibres
The idea is to encourage—not deter—you from making the most of what you've got. Many competitors reach the top by breaking the rules. There *are* short basketball players and skinny javelin throwers, but they are successful because they possess extra mental competitive qualities that, as yet, cannot be measured.

They will also have the right balance of muscle fibres. Internally, muscular factors decide how well we do at sport. Each muscle is made up of two sorts of fibres: *fast twitch* for explosive, split-second power—eg, sprinting, weight-lifting, hitting a tennis smash; *slow twitch* for endurance—eg, long-distance running, cycling, swimming. These keep us going a long time.

Each of us is born with a fixed proportion of fast and slow twitch muscle fibres, but we can make sure that we get the best out of each type by using the right sort of training. Though you can never be a successful marathon runner if you have a preponderance of the sprinter's fast twitch muscles, or a successful sprinter if you have mostly slow twitch fibres.

Your Dominant Muscle Fibre: If you are good at catching a bus (sprinting over a short distance) then you may have more fast twitch fibres. If you enjoy a long walk (45 minutes—1 hour) with no ill-effects, then the endurance-type slow twitch may make up your main muscle structure.

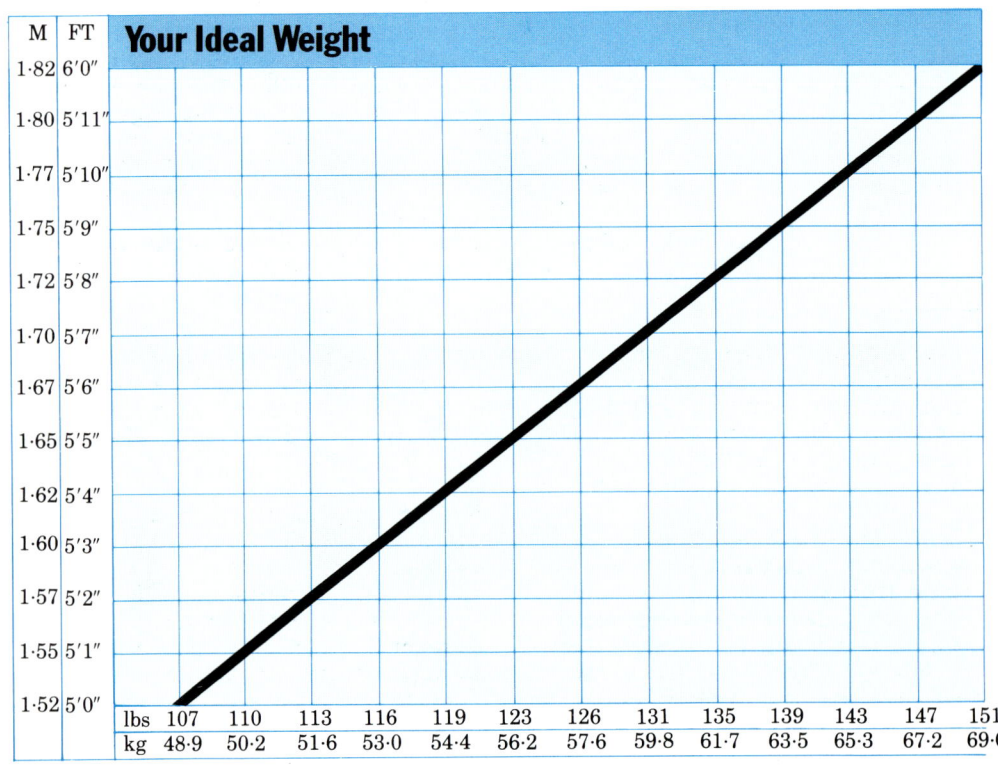
Your Ideal Weight

STARTING TO EXERCISE

Body Shape and Sport

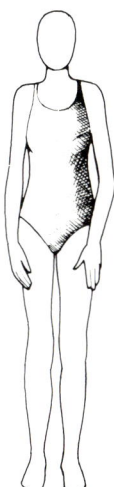 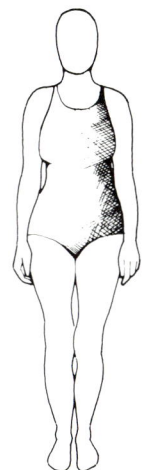 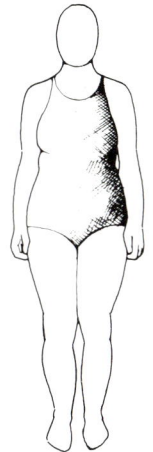

Ectomorph: This is the thin extreme of the spectrum; tall, lanky, skinny. Lightweight—well-suited to marathon running. No good at throwing or rowing or sports where strength is important.

Mesomorph: The happy medium— not too skinny, not too broad, but may tend towards putting on weight easily. Good all rounders, likely to do reasonably well at anything that combines spurts of speed with endurance—eg, squash, badminton, tennis matches.

Endomorph: Well endowed with subcutaneous fat; not able to do much on dry land apart from cycling —but benefits greatly from buoyancy in water to enjoy swimming (especially long distance); this is extreme, there are few natural endomorphs.

Ectomorphic-Mesomorph: A mixture of thin and muscular. Athletic: good at running, jumping, combining agility and strength. A base-line tennis player, a good badminton player, and gymnast.

Endomorphic-Mesomorph: Moving towards the tubby end of the scale, this is a familiar figure, and often a successful athlete although with a tendency to gain weight. Suits aggressive sports because of built-in power and protection— downhill skiing, cricket (bowling), softball (pitching), volleyball (setter). If tall, good at basketball, volleyball; if short, good at sprinting and some field events like shotputt, discus throwing.

Ectomorphic-Endomorph: A seemingly weird combination of the extremes of the spectrum that is quite common: large-hipped, large-busted ladies. Sport is rarely their forte, but this may be the result of social conditioning; they benefit from keep-fit, dance and yoga-type routines.

29

Preparation

Wear the Right Gear

Before you get started it is worth your while to invest in some proper sportswear. This will not only boost your morale and encourage you to take your fitness and exercise programme seriously, but also help ensure that you are comfortable and unhampered while working out, as reputable manufacturers never forget that these clothes have a job to do once you start moving

First and foremost, wear the right shoes as the many bones in your feet, your ankles, knees and hips all need support, protection and cushioning. Second, buy a sports bra. Even if you do not normally wear a bra, you will appreciate the support and comfort a sports bra affords when working out. If necessary, buy two for different times of the month—a supporting bra isn't much good if it is too tight. (If you are pregnant, see p. 73.) Third, if you want to wear socks choose short, cotton ones which will allow your feet to 'breathe' and won't constrict the veins in your calves. Fourth, buy comfortable and suitable clothes. For dance and stretching, choose comfortably-fitting leotards. These should be well-contoured but not constricting in any way. The ones which are made of cotton (90%) and elasticated fibre (10%) are best as they move with you, keep you both cool and warm and allow your skin to breathe. For running, jogging, cycling and walking in summer, wear shorts, lightweight sleeved or sleeveless T-shirt (or cool cotton trousers for brisk walking). In the autumn and winter, you will benefit by wearing tracksuit bottoms to keep your legs warm. This will prevent your body from expending valuable energy just to keep you warm. T-shirts and tracksuit tops or sweat shirts are very convenient between seasons. Once you're well and truly warmed up during your workout, you can slip off your top and tie the arms around your waist.

Always choose cottons or cotton mixtures: they wash well, absorb sweat, allow your skin to breathe and keep you both warm and cool.

Shoes

Research into how to protect the foot during exercise—which in turn protects the leg and back—has transformed the thin-soled gym shoe or sneaker into a bouncy, thick-soled shock absorber for the 21 bones in each foot. But what shoe should you buy and how much should you spend? Here are some tips:

Buy the right shoes for the job: Joggers need different shoes from tennis players; an aerobic dancer needs something that a basketball player would never wear. Therefore, go to a specialist shop where the sales people are often participants and spend time with them, trying on what they suggest. Take your time.

Advertising: Don't go for the shoe you saw advertised most on TV, it

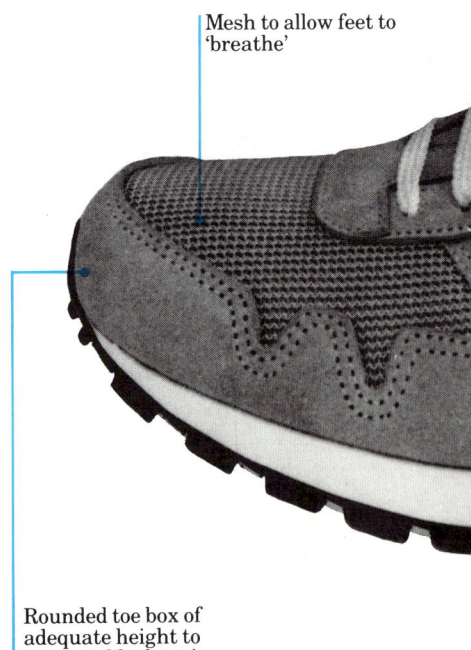

Mesh to allow feet to 'breathe'

Rounded toe box of adequate height to prevent 'black toe'

STARTING TO EXERCISE

might not suit your needs. What's more, the shoe you saw an Olympic running champion wearing was designed to run fast in and won't have the sort of support the average runner needs.

Price: The basic rule of thumb is not to buy anything too cheap because you'll get less wear and tear for your money, and the shoes will be less well designed. On the other hand, don't feel you must buy the most expensive shoes either.

Orthotics: These are shoe inserts that correct the angle at which your foot hits the ground. You will often see people with shoes (both casual and sporty) that are heavily worn on one side. If this is the result of the foot rolling outwards excessively, they are over 'supinating', if it's the result of their foot rolling inwards, then this is over 'pronating'. Both can be corrected by orthotics. If you have shoes that wear like this, show them to the shop assistants. It will help in purchasing the right shoe.

Achilles tendon protectors: These tabs at the heel of the shoes are specially designed to protect your Achilles tendon. However in some instances these can irritate the Achilles tendon. If this occurs, purchase shoes which do not have heel tabs.

Breaking shoes in: Wear your new shoes, loosely laced, about the house for a few hours each day to break them in before using them for your workout.

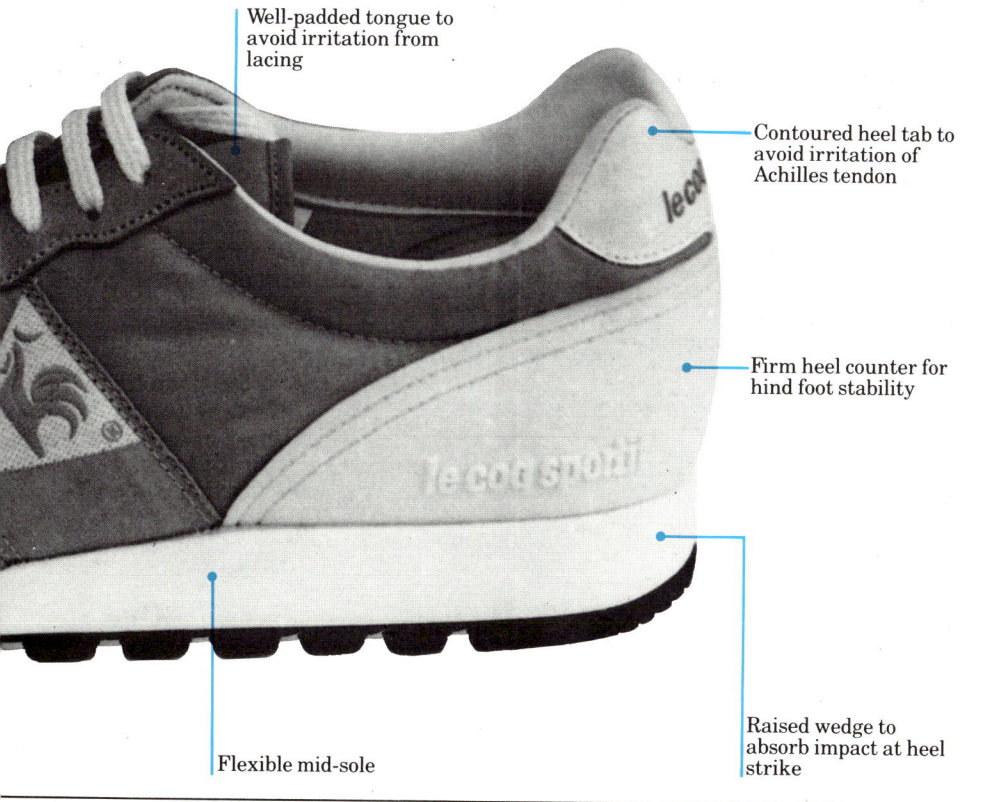

Well-padded tongue to avoid irritation from lacing

Contoured heel tab to avoid irritation of Achilles tendon

Firm heel counter for hind foot stability

Flexible mid-sole

Raised wedge to absorb impact at heel strike

STARTING TO EXERCISE

Pacing Yourself

Exercise affects us all differently. You might be the same age, height, weight and build as someone else but may get fitter, faster or slower. However, the need to break yourself in gently and gradually cannot be emphasised enough especially if you haven't exercised for a while. Of course there will be some *aches* at first, but you should not have to suffer *pain*. That is a sign of over-doing it. In fact, the slower the build up, the more thorough it is and the longer the benefits will last.

Targets

There is nothing more depressing than watching people work out because 'it's good for me, because I'll live longer'. Exercise has to be enjoyable, has to be fun, and ideally, should be something shared between friends and family. People who take the attitude that exercise is imperative for their own good risk becoming exercise addicts—and they are no fun to be around. However, we all thrive on achievement: at home, at school, at work. With a target to aim at, exercise can be equally rewarding. It could be as simple as completing a local fun run, playing in a club tennis tournament, or going for a hike with your kids. Many women who have felt little or no sense of achievement in their lives, find that exercise and sport suddenly fulfils ambitions that were only ignited by a realisation of their own physical potential. So pick a target—a modest one at first—and once you've done that, move up another step.

Basic Exercise Plan

Walking

This is something most of us do every day. However, it is largely ignored as a form of exercise because it's too easy. Walking is excellent, working the body's major muscles, and is boosted if you swing your arms enthusiastically too.

What to Wear: No special clothing is needed, but as with most sports, comfortable shock-absorbing shoes with good cotton socks are vital. Wear layers of clothing, so that if you work up a bit of a sweat you can remove a thin top layer without getting chilled.

Where to Walk and How Fast: The point about using walking as exercise is to *go somewhere*. A stroll round the block is certainly a start, but a target is always a great help. If you have no 'circuit', walk for 10 minutes (don't guess, look at your watch, time will go by slowly), then turn round and come home so that you don't overdo it. Eventually, you should aim for a brisk pace which goes non-stop for about 30–40 minutes. This will raise your pulse rate and get your circulation going. If you can work out a circuit of about a mile and cover that once, if not twice a day, you will feel the benefits more quickly than you imagine. But don't dither and dawdle, stop and chat or do the shopping as well. You can't enjoy a brisk walk *and* carry a shopping bag.

Keeping It Up: Although many women might consider jogging or running as the next step up, it is a pity to neglect walking as serious exercise in its own right. Rambling, long distance walking, hiking and orienteering (see p. 146) are excellent for both body and soul, particularly if going through the countryside and over hills and dales.

Competitive race walking, however, is an unnatural form of exercise with a high risk of injury.

Jogging and Running

The idea of running to get fit has taken a surprisingly long time to catch on—several thousand years in fact. Some argue that the trendy name 'jogging' persuaded people that they were doing something totally new. In many ways they were. What most of us had to do at least once at school was boring, embarrassing, painful and futile. Jogging is no longer boring because it is 'new' and a few precious moments alone can be relaxing. As so many people jog, it is more accepted and less embarrassing. Modern shoes and careful adherence to proper warm-up and stretching, built into a graduated programme has eliminated much of the

Warm Up Properly

Top class athletes spend as much as an hour getting their bodies and minds together before a big event. That is one extreme. However, the other extreme—of doing nothing—is asking for trouble. Wriggle your fingers and toes, flex your ankles and wrists, shake out your arms and legs, roll your shoulders, pitter-patter lightly on your feet, get your blood circulating, get your heart rate up a little, let the oxygen get to all parts of the body before asking it to do anything. Then—and only then—go into a gentle stretching routine.

pain. And as running does us good, it is no longer futile. As for the weather, that depends where you live. However, in the main, we live indoor lives, and every experience of the outdoors, wet or dry, hot or cold, can be invigorating.

Do run or jog at your own pace. Psychiatrist Kenneth E Callen decided that the most obvious differences between 424 female and male first-time runners were that 'Women tended to start running to lose weight, while competition attracted large numbers of men. More women feel creative while running, while men are more apt to picture themselves winning races.'

What to Wear: One reason for running or jogging's popularity is its low cost: no rackets or balls, nets or courts are needed. However, good shoes are essential (see p. 30). Complement these with absorbent cotton socks and loose comfortable clothing. Jeans are impractical because they tend to rub and retain the heat too much. In warm weather shorts and a running vest or T-shirt is fine, but in cooler weather be sure to wear a loose, well-designed tracksuit. If your heart has to pump out more blood to keep your legs warm, it is doing extra work, and it is always easy to take off a layer if you get too hot.

Where to Run: You can run anywhere. That is its appeal. However, there are some places that are better than others. If you start out on nothing but the hard surfaces of roads, pavement and sidewalks, then your legs will suffer, however good the shock absorbers in your running shoes. Try to run on grass as much as possible; get out into the park or better, into the countryside. Many towns have jogging trails which are worth following, as well as being a good place to meet fellow joggers. Never ignore the social and psychological benefits of sport, where sharing the fun and frustration can be so rewarding.

Running on sand is often an attraction on vacation. However, that open expanse by the tideline can be very hard, especially if you run barefoot. It can make your ankles and knees feel very sore afterwards. Likewise, the soft sand higher up the beach can give unfit leg muscles and stiff ligaments and tendons a tortuous workout, stretching them more than you realise (especially the Achilles tendon), until you wake up stiff and sore the next day. So be careful not to get carried away and start up exercise too enthusiastically on holiday!

How Fast?: Putting one foot in front of another seems simple enough, but it's well worth remembering that the speed that your arms go backwards and forwards can govern the speed of your legs. Try it when you are walking. Isn't it easier to swing your arms?

If you have done nothing in the way of exercise for some time, start slowly. Very slowly. In fact, the best thing to do is to walk 100 yards and jog 100 yards. Pick out a tree or a bench or a lamp post—walk to it, jog to the next. Take it gently. Once you get jogging, relax your shoulders, let your arms swing loosely, elbows bent, hands also held loosely and, most important, with your mouth relaxed. Gritting your teeth tenses up your neck muscles and can make you tense your shoulders. Try smiling, running with your mouth slightly open. Take reasonable steps: don't be a tippy-toed fairy, don't take great strides. Look for a comfortable, happy medium. As for speed, do the 'talk test'—just talk to yourself or your companion. If you are going too fast, you won't be able to . . . so the 'talk test' ensures that you aren't

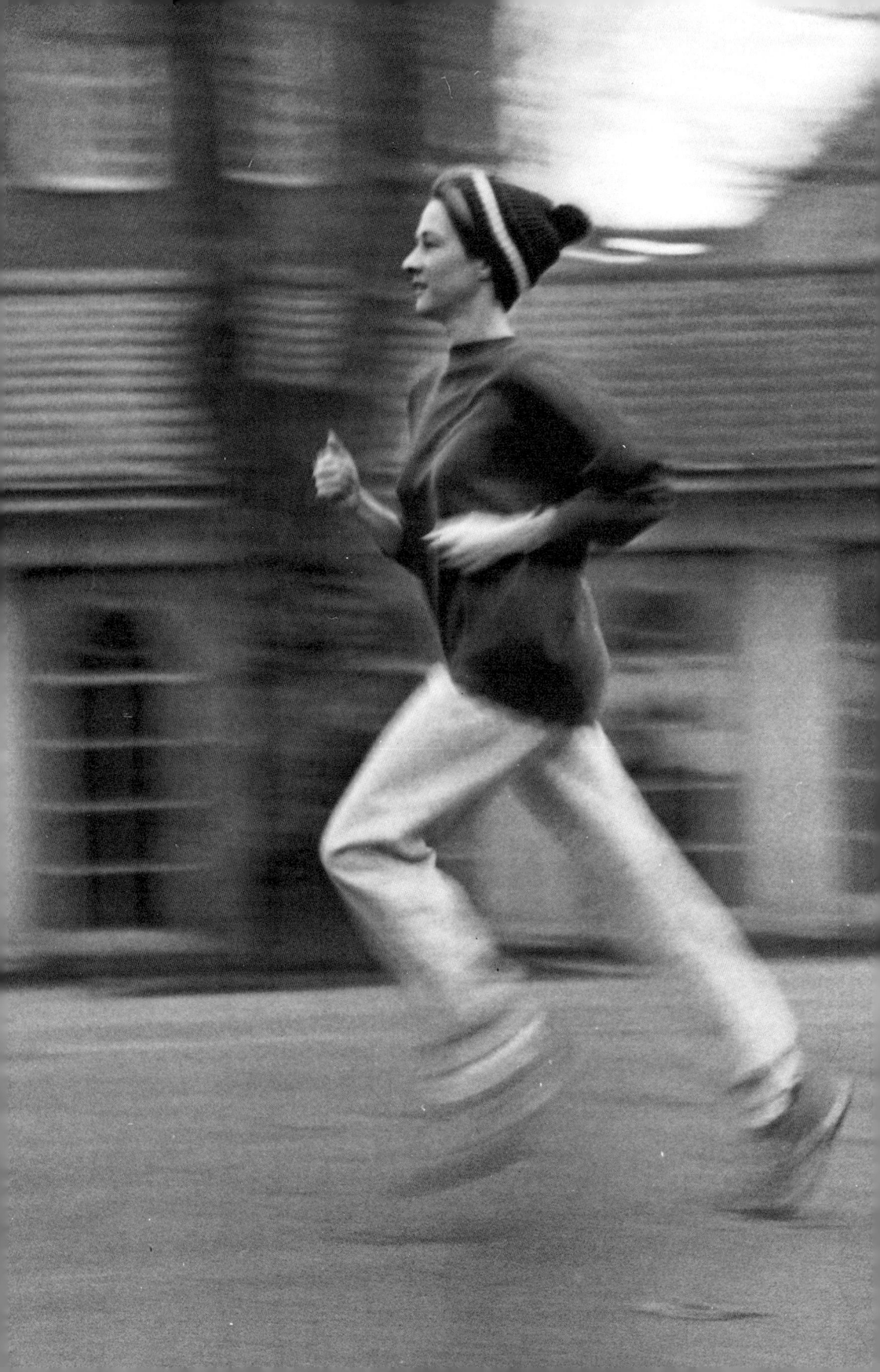

overdoing it. Early on, this may be barely faster than walking pace!

Keeping It Up: You should get a big round of applause for starting up, but after a while no one is encouraging you any more. After all, starting is the hard part. However, after a few weeks, most people suddenly feel that they're getting nowhere, that there is no sense of achievement. This can be overcome in several ways.

First, as we've said, companionship is a great help: you can egg each other on, and by fixing dates together, you won't want to let the other down.

Secondly, make a note in your diary of what your body is up to: *your weight*—it may drop—which won't do any harm—but quite often it stays constant as fat turns to muscle; *your pulse rate*—it should drop as you get fitter; *time spent running*—don't get competitive about this, just work out regularly. Later log *distances and times*—so that you get the satisfaction of improvement. But don't do a personal best every night.

Third, set yourself a target. With so many organised events available over specific distances, aim to enter one in a few months time. Don't make this the London or New York marathon. So few entries are accepted you could be disappointed, and anyway, a marathon, however inspiring and romantic, is not a reasonable target. Go for a community event, or a series of events.

If you get really carried away by running as an exercise-style on its own —fine!—although you could add variety to your workouts by making it a *part* of an all-round plan or try orienteering (see p. 146). You may meet or have read about women who are 'hooked' on running. Scientists have discovered that the serenity—and even euphoria—experienced by runners is caused by hormone-like chemicals in the brain. These 'endorphins' not only make you feel good, but also help you eat *less*—unless you actually need more food. Meanwhile, the so-called 'runners high' is reckoned to assist top-class athletes through exhausting and even painful training.

Swimming

There is little doubt that swimming is regarded as the most desirable form of exercise by the experts. It uses all the large muscle groups (especially round the shoulders, stomach and bottom), it produces little or no wear and tear, few, if any, injuries and can be fun. It builds stamina, strengthens the heart and lungs, and aids flexibility. The only drawbacks are the inconvenience—if there is no nearby pool—and the fact that many adults don't know how to swim, or if they swim well, find the pools jampacked when they want to swim 'lengths'.

If you are an adult who cannot swim, don't be embarrassed about using the same aids as children: inflatable armbands, rubber rings etc. Once you have your legs working well, the arm action will follow. Start off by enjoying yourself; fitness will come later. If you had a bad experience trying to swim as a child, tell an instructor who may be able to help you overcome this psychological stumbling block and avoid trying to learn to swim with children.

What to Wear: Wear a swimsuit for swimming and keep your bikini for sunbathing only. Not only is an all-in-one unlikely to fall off or come apart when you dive or jump in, but it will also keep you warmer by offering better insulation.

Nylon-lycra suits are best because they offer a two-way stretch and are more comfortable and flattering than cotton-lycra or all-nylon suits. There are many different styles of swimsuit available; you should try these on and buy whichever feels most comfortable. Most are cut high on the leg nowadays for maximum movement. Some of the newer styles incorporate the 'Super Fly Back' cut. These have no vertical seams and so eliminate air pockets and fit very snugly to the contours of your body.

Goggles: These are strongly recommended to protect your eyes from chlorine. They also improve your vision underwater. If you are allergic to the rubber surrounds, hypo-allergenic goggles are also available.

Caps: These are also recommended, not only to protect your hair from the drying and bleaching ravages of

STARTING TO EXERCISE

Pool Exercises
For Stomach Muscles

1 Standing in shoulder-depth water, grasp side of pool and keep trunk vertical against wall. Lift legs and hold straight at right-angles to trunk. Use stomach muscles to keep legs from sinking.

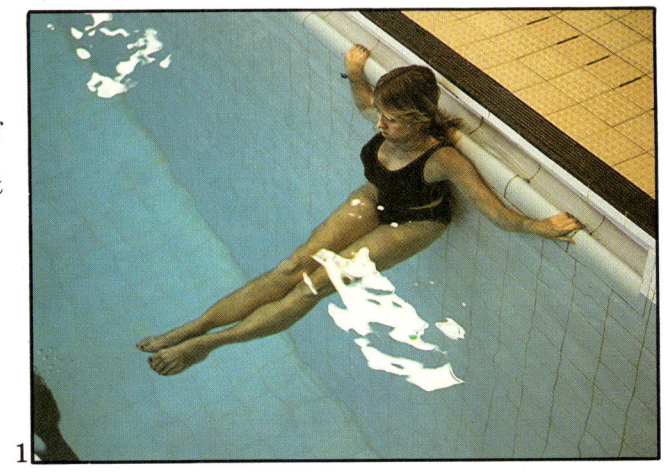

2 Grasping side of pool, stretch body out straight, then swing legs gently from waist to left and right, using stomach muscles to keep legs afloat. Repeat 15 times.

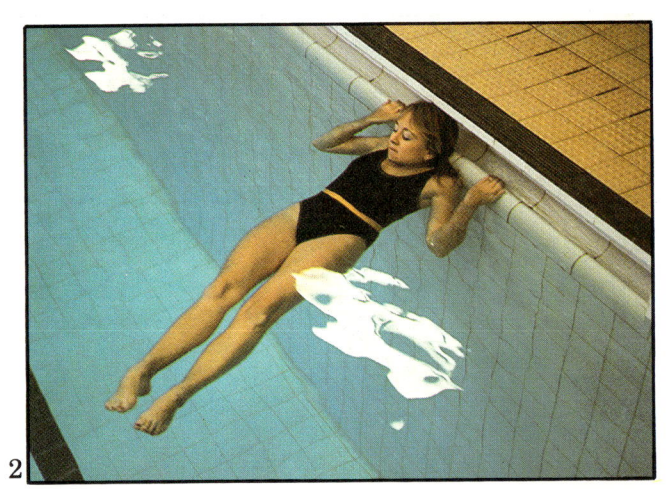

3 As above, but cross right leg over left and vice-versa while keeping upper body still and legs afloat.

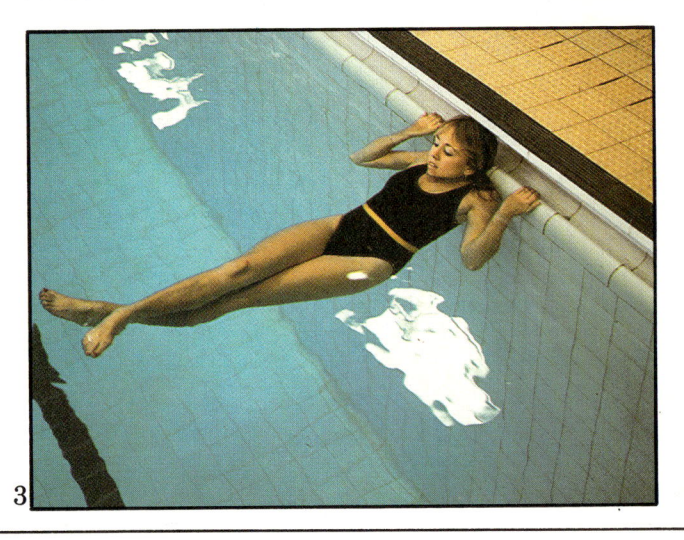

STARTING TO EXERCISE

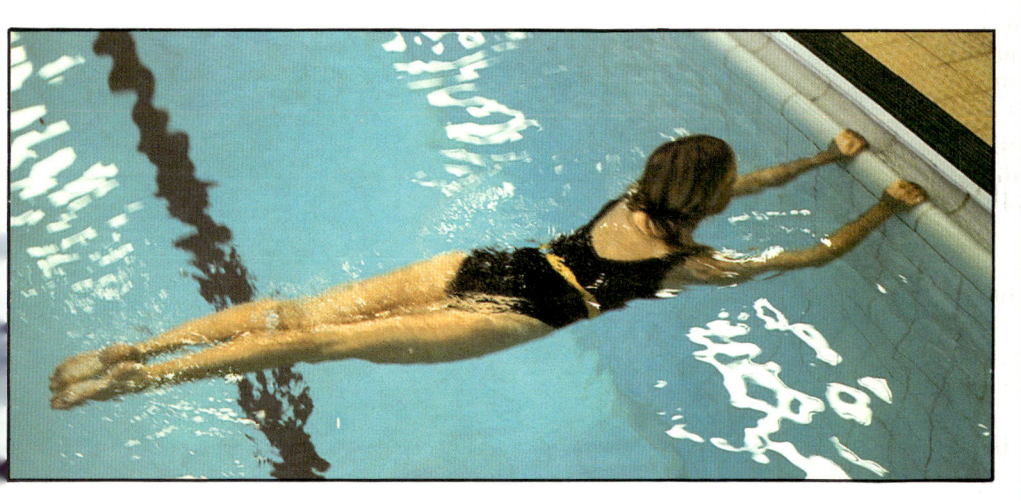

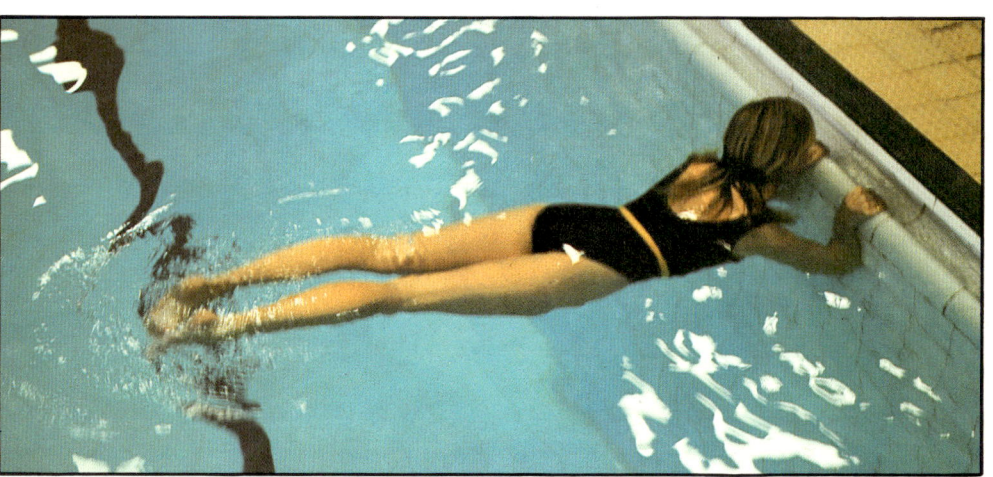

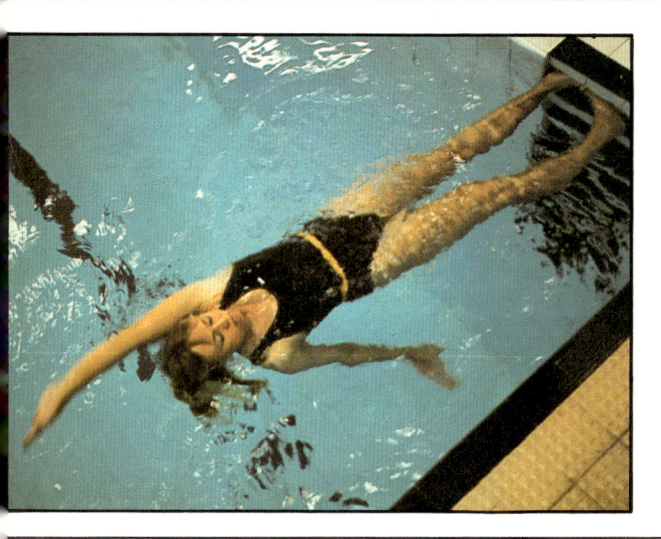

For Arms and Shoulders

4 & 5 Floating on front with arms and legs extended, bend arms at elbow to pull body to side of pool. When head reaches wall, straighten and extend arms. Repeat 10 times.

6 Lie on back, hooking toes under bar at poolside. (If no bar hook heel over 'gutter'). Do back crawl arm movements, thrusting arms deep into the water.

37

chlorine, but also for safety and so that you can see where you are going!

Where to Swim: Swimming pools are the best place to learn to swim. Once you are competent and know you won't panic, you can swim in pools, rivers, lakes, the sea—there are no limits as long as the water is clean and the beach safe. Do check lakes and oceans where pollution is becoming a bigger problem, especially in the Mediterranean and on the shores of many developing countries where sewage is poured directly into the water. Check currents and tides, and supervise children *at all times*, as accidents can happen in seconds. Drowning is the biggest recreational killer for children, and kids ought to be taught to swim properly as soon as possible. The sea and rivers are high risk areas for youngsters.

How Fast?: Unlike running, swimming is very difficult to overdo unless you swim out to the middle of a lake or out to sea and get too exhausted to return. In a pool, a target time should be set—see Basic Schedule and Workout Plans—although for real effect, at least 30 yards per minute should be covered. If you finish in the allotted time feeling fresh, don't go on, but step up your pace slightly *next time*.

There are four strokes and each has physical benefits: *crawl*—develops naturally from the beginner's doggy paddle; good for stomach, arms, shoulders, legs and at full tilt is good for heart and lungs; *backstroke*—good for upper arms, flexibility; *butterfly*—good for strengthening shoulders, but can give lower back problems; *breaststroke* —the hardest to perfect but good for the upper arms, chest, inner thigh and pelvic floor.

Keeping It Up: The problem with swimming is that covering lap after lap of a pool can get very boring. So we suggest that you combine swimming with exercises in the water. The resistance of the water is a great way to tone up your muscles. These are especially useful if you only have the use of a small pool, where flat-out swimming is either impossible or frustratingly brief from wall to wall.

Cycling

The advantages of cycling over many other sports are now being recognised —particularly in the USA where it rose to second most popular recreation by 1985. In countries like Denmark, the bicycle has been a popular mode of travel for decades—more a way of life than a way of keeping fit. Where cycling scores over running and jogging is that it does not put stress on to the knee and ankle joints as long as the saddle height is properly adjusted; something to remember if you sustain a running injury. If you are particularly overweight, it is a good form of exercise to start out with—perhaps in combination with swimming—because your extra weight could otherwise stress your lower limbs. Cycling is great for older women too as they tend to have more brittle bones and can greatly benefit from the effort of pedalling, which strengthens bones. Cycling is also a sociable, family activity.

What to Ride: Like cars and driving, it is important that the bicycle you ride is in good working order. So, think twice before venturing out on an old rusty bicycle that hasn't been used for years. First, your bicycle must be the right frame size: too big and you risk a nasty accident, too small and you'll quickly get pain in the knee joint. Handlebars, whether straight or 'drop', should be at the right height and arms' length. You also need a comfortable saddle. Most are made of plastic and foam nowadays and are comfortable but give less wear and tear than leather ones. Leather saddles take a lot of breaking in but eventually, as they are moulded to your contours, you don't even notice they're there! Equally important is that you have reachable, effective back and front brakes, back and front lights, sound tyres with good treads, and somewhere on the bike to put your possessions— never sling anything across the handlebars or your shoulder, it upsets the centre of gravity and therefore your balance. You also need gears—just like a car does. Three is the minimum, but you can go for five, ten, or twelve depending on where and how much you intend to cycle.

While you need not rush out and buy

STARTING TO EXERCISE

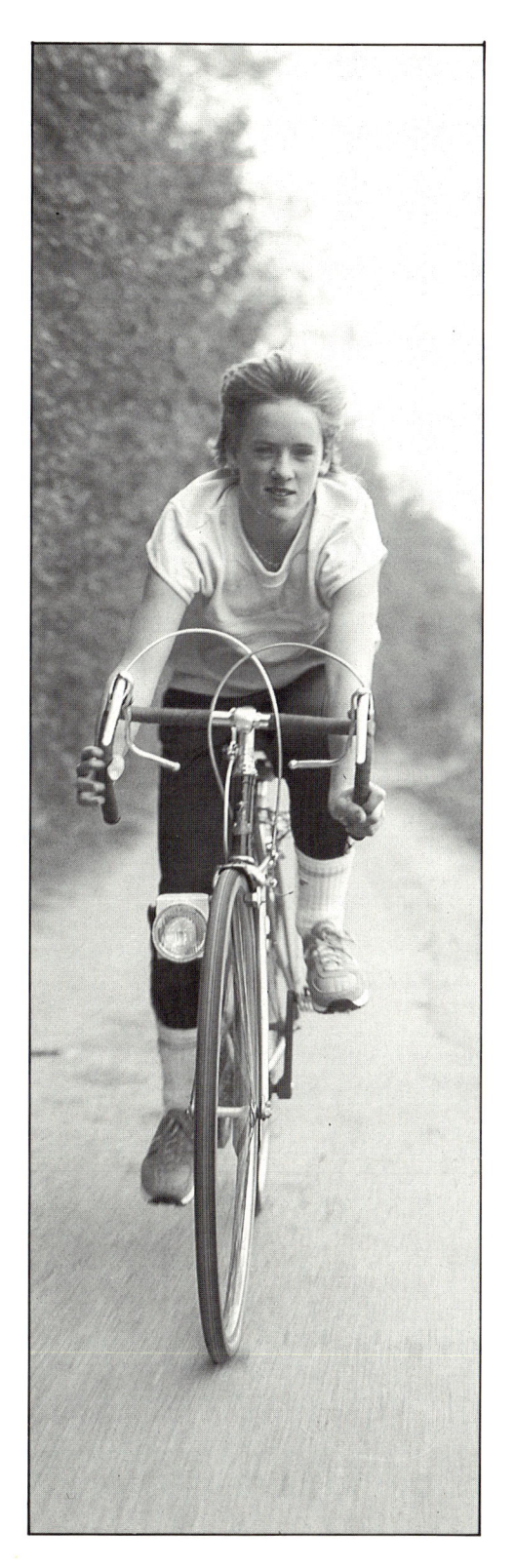

the latest racing model, do bear in mind that if you envisage *any* town cycling you must have good tyre treads, brakes and gears. These are essential: to keep you moving, make you stop and enable you to get out of the way quickly. It is no good having fast reflexes if your bicycle cannot or will not respond to your commands.

What to Wear: If you are taking up cycling as a serious form of exercise, covering more than five miles each day, then it is well worth investing in the proper protective gear—shorts fitted with chamois leather crotch pieces. These are comfortable and very effective. If, on the other hand cycling is merely a fit way of getting about town, then you'll be just as comfortable in sweat-absorbing cotton shorts (with tracksuit bottoms in chilly weather) along with loose-fitting sweat tops. Special gloves, hats and cycle shoes are optional extras unless you are earnest about cycling and plan to cover distances. Wear layers of clothing so that you are prepared to add or subtract depending on your body temperature and the wind.

Where to Cycle: The major drawback about cycling is safety. Where the automobile is king, the cyclist is very vulnerable. Special cycle paths are more and more popular, but we cannot emphasise enough the importance of sticking to the highway code, being extra vigilant wherever you go and making sure you are seen. Make sure your brakes and your lights work effectively. Keep your eyes skinned and *never* take risks in built-up areas. On the other hand, quiet lanes ignored by cars are often surprisingly common and local cycle clubs are experts on good routes.

In bad weather indoor exercise bikes can build up your heart and lungs and legs quite well, but the upper part of your body (which gets some exercise outdoors as it helps balance you on your bike) gets little or no benefit indoors. Exercise bikes can also become rather boring—fitting into the 'I'm doing it because it does me good' ethic. However, if you cannot face going out to cycle, they can be a distinct bonus, though you

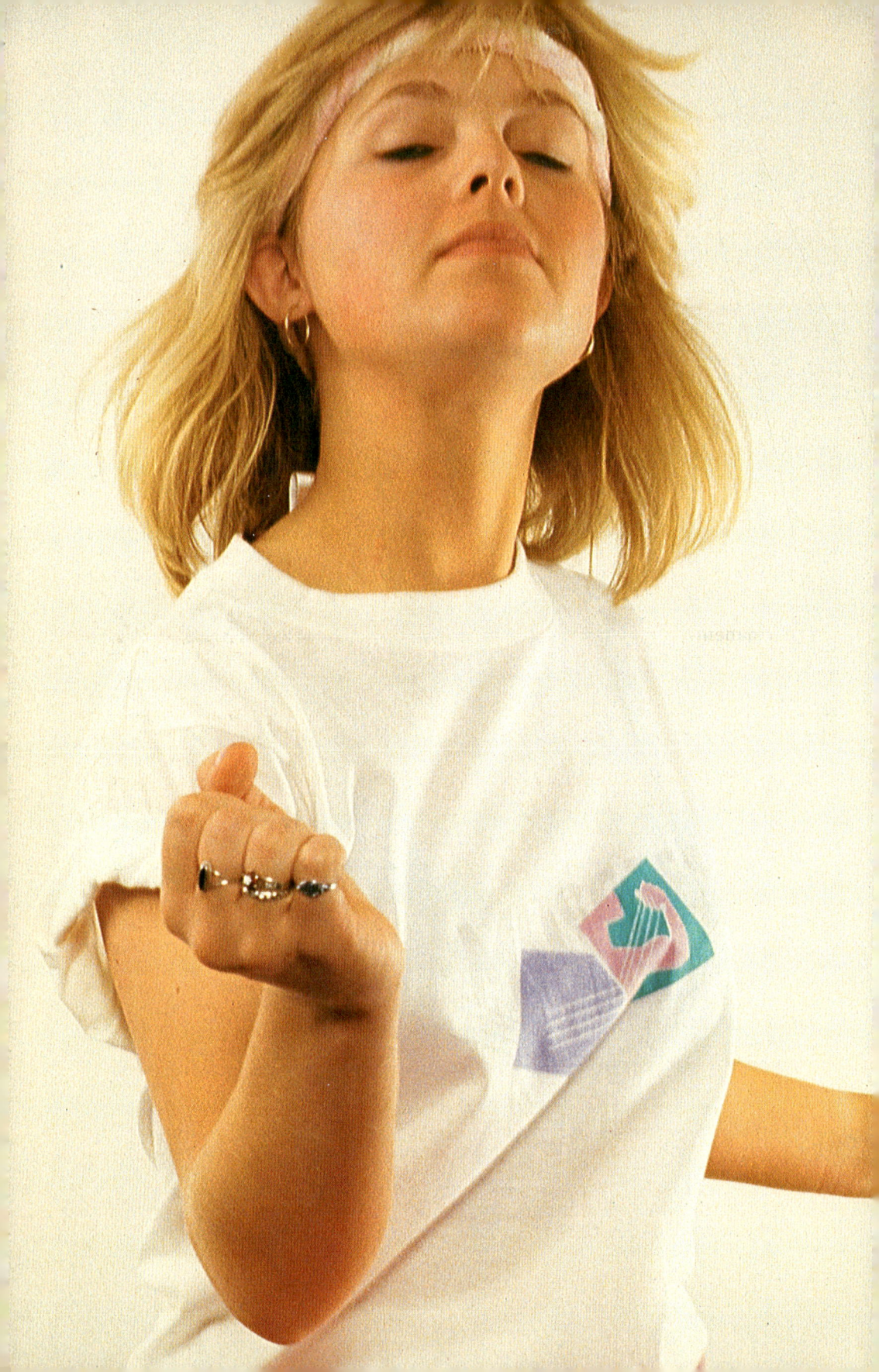

STARTING TO EXERCISE

shouldn't ignore the invigorating 'back to nature' feeling of cycling in the rain —as long as you have the right rainproof gear on!

How Fast?: Cycling is useful because you can use the gears to help you work out. At first, the lowest gear makes cycling easy and lets your muscles ease into the idea of exercise. As you spend more time in the saddle, push the gears up, making it harder for yourself. Eventually, you will be able to use the highest gear in short bursts as a form of training, but for long distances low gears are more appropriate.

Just as we recommend a 'talk test' for joggers and runners, so the same criterion applies to cycling. As long as you can chat and talk aloud as you cycle you are not overdoing it—but be careful about cycling abreast! As you cycle, keep everything relaxed even though you are watching the road. Start with your mouth and jaw, and continue down your neck and shoulders. Many cyclists are permanently tense because they grip the handlebars too tightly. Make sure you are in the correct position.

Keeping It Up: One attraction of cycling is that you can get somewhere quite quickly and easily, so targets can be set and met. Cycle to see friends, to the pub (stick to soft drinks—drinking and cycling is dangerous), or the shops. Join a cycling club so that you can join in a longer ride at weekends. A vacation on a bicycle is a wonderful way for a family to have fun, and that can also act as a target. In France the local railroad stations hire out bicycles—and similar schemes operate in many countries round the world.

Dance

This is one of the most natural and ancient forms of movement and self-expression. It may be fast and assertive, or slow, graceful and sensuous, or highly rhythmical. While dance obviously uses the muscles in the legs and feet, the arms, head, neck, and hip joint are also involved—the stomach muscles too, particularly in oriental-type belly-dancing. Dance can give you a very high degree of fitness and stamina (ballet dancing) or just the benefit of an occasional workout. Stretching exercises are usually a feature of all forms of dance, and while good posture may not be a prerequisite to begin with, it is quickly acquired.

Many highly organised systems of music and movement have been around for years and are well worth investigating. For example the Margaret Morris Movement (MMM)

Aerobics

Aerobic means 'with oxygen', the opposite of *anaerobic* (without oxygen). Aerobic exercise was advocated by an American doctor called Kenneth H Cooper who pointed out that an efficient heart/lung system, one that could convert the air you breathe into energy easily, was the basis of a healthy life. He then said that jogging, cycling, swimming and walking were the best way of giving you what we commonly call 'stamina'. In other words, he believed in sports that took a long time to do at a reasonably slow pace, where you need to breathe in and out steadily. *Anaerobic* exercise is the opposite: it is the explosive power needed for sports like sprinting and weightlifting.

Unfortunately, many so-called 'aerobics' classes encourage physical jerks, where you need a big breath to make a quick movement, and this is actually *anaerobic*. The main problem with aerobics classes is that while they may be led or taught by women who are super-fit, their system very often does not allow enough warm-up before a session, let alone a gradual build-up for newcomers. However, these classes, when they are properly taught, are ideal for *keeping* you fit, but not *getting* you fit.

STARTING TO EXERCISE

was 75 years old in 1985. A child prodigy and ballet dancer, Margaret Morris drew on traditional forms of exercise like Greek dance (from Isadora Duncan's brother) and Hatha Yoga. Her system of recreational dance emphasises breathing with all the exercises, mobility of the spine and opposition of the arms and legs. In its simplest form, it is a type of physical fitness routine, but has the added benefits of being educational by developing our creative and aesthetic qualities. By setting targets, adherents work their way through a series of grades (named after colours) which at the top level are tough enough to challenge expert gymnasts or dancers.

What to Wear: As with all other forms of exercise, a good warm-up before you begin is crucial in the prevention of injury. Many dancers like to stretch and warm-up with an extra layer over their leotards and there are many cotton or cotton-mixture tops available. Muscles work better when they are warm, so legwarmers on top of dance tights are a must at the beginning of your dance session even though the studio might be well heated. In order to dance well and allow for as much unrestricted movement as possible, a shallow cut leotard with a high cut-away leg is the most comfortable. Both dance tights and leotard should fit as snugly as possible for maximum body definition and comfort.

Although most dance classes will advocate bare feet, there is a risk of injury. Research at San Diego State University has shown that in a ten-minute spell of all-out exercise, each foot can hit the floor as many as one thousand times! Add the full weight of the body crashing down each time and you'll see why the bare foot with its complex structure of bones and muscles has a huge task, especially if you are just starting up. There are special shoes now available to help the woman who does dance or keep fit and these are specifically designed to do the right job, like an athlete's shoes. Running shoes or trainers are not right for the job as they tend to protect the heel (used in running) and to be flat (to counteract sideways motion).

Basic Exercise Plan

These five types of exercise have been worked into a weekly routine that has been adapted for all age groups and used successfully by teenagers through to seventy and eighty year olds. There are three sections each day:

Pattering, one of the simplest and most effective fitness exercises.

Stretching, again a simple but effective muscle toner.

Basic exercise, your own choice and combination of walking, jogging, swimming, cycling and dance.

Each plan is designed for a specific age group:

Plan One—15–25 years

Plan Two—25–35 years

Plan Three—35–50 years

Plan Four—50 years and over

But all are based on one idea—*daily* pattering and stretching. Each day, a couple of minutes (at the most) is spent pattering (opposite). This is followed by 2 or 3 minutes of stretching. Your week can begin whenever you like, depending on your free time. Then utilise whichever basic exercises you prefer for your workout and slot them into the timetable. We believe that *consecutive* days of exercise are more beneficial than the usual one day on, one day off. That is why there are two days off at a time on our charts. However, we expect you to spend 5 minutes pattering and stretching on these days, even if you don't go swimming or dancing; everyone has 5 minutes to spare!

There is one golden rule: *take your time*. We have deliberately started each plan with as little as 5 minutes exercise a day. Many women are put off further workouts by the agonies and aches brought on by overdoing it. Please, take it easy. If you feel on top of the world after a few weeks, then increase the intensity of your exercise. Don't increase the time spent on exercising.

These exercises can be done at any time. Some of us feel great in the morning and feel that it is the only time to work out. Others have to wait until lunch break or the evening—especially if there are children to look after. If you always feel sluggish at one time of day, try a different time—you might find it easier and more enjoyable. After you exercise, remember to warm down or cool down. Just as you take time to get in gear before exertions, let your body down gently afterwards. Stretch a little and then shake out your arms and legs to encourage the circulation to carry away the body's waste products (mainly lactic acid).

Tips for Success

- **Discipline yourself**
  Stick to your workout plan and stick to the part of the day and the length of time you have allocated yourself. Don't let anyone or anything cheat you or beguile you into skipping a session.

- **Work hard**
  Work out properly—to a sweat-raising pulse. Go for quality rather than quantity, but preferably go for both:
  10 minutes cycling is better than 20 minutes dawdling, but 15 minutes brisk walking is better than either!

- **Make time**
  Work out how long it will take you to get changed, patter, stretch, workout, warm down, shower and dress, then double it and put aside the time. Get into the habit of making this time a special part of the day when you're doing something entirely for yourself.

- **Be patient**
  People who give up after only a short time usually do so because they have put in too much, too soon. Train but don't strain; fitness is about fun not pain.

Pattering

The simplest part of the Basic Exercise Plan is also the most effective as well as being the least time consuming.

Called *Pattering*, it was invented by Gordon Richards MBE in 1956 and has helped him to train World and Olympic champions in a dozen sports.

The Idea
It *looks* like running on the spot but it isn't.

- you run quickly on your toes
- your feet barely leave the ground
- you do *not* lift your knees
- you must make sure your arms and legs are co-ordinated, even as you quicken the pace

The Result
Pattering is remarkably tiring when done correctly. You 'feel' it after a matter of seconds, so no session is longer than 2 minutes!

The Benefits
- Increases your heart's strength
- Increases efficiency of your lungs
- Increases your speed of reaction
- Strengthens your legs but, unlike jogging or running, does NOT stress the knee and ankle joints.

There will be a noticeable tightening of the calf muscle (at the back of lower leg) after the first few days. This will soon go away. There are two speeds recommended by Mr Richards—slow and fast. In combination, they give you a first-class workout.

Slow Patter—is still pretty quick, almost too quick to count! However, it's about 50 steps in 10 seconds. Now you can understand why it is so demanding.

Fast Patter—as fast as you can, remembering that your arms must still work in co-ordination with your legs.

STARTING TO EXERCISE

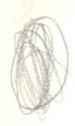

Stretching

Try the following, remembering to press gently into the tension, hold it at the edge of discomfort, and then relax gently. *Do not bounce!* Enthusiastic women on TV shows may do physical jerks in their earnestness to impress you and keep in time to the music, but *do not imitate them*! That jerkiness can cause injury, while it is only holding the stretch for several seconds that does you any good at all. But don't hold your breath—breathe in and out evenly as you stretch and relax.

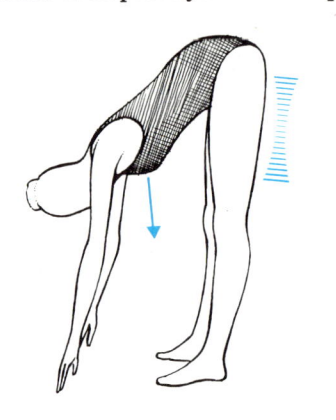

1 Hamstring Stretch
Stretches injury-prone hamstring muscle at back of thigh.
Keep legs straight and comfortably apart. Keep back straight, bend from waist and reach forward with arms hanging loosely. Don't flop down: this is not a quick 'touch the toes' exercise.

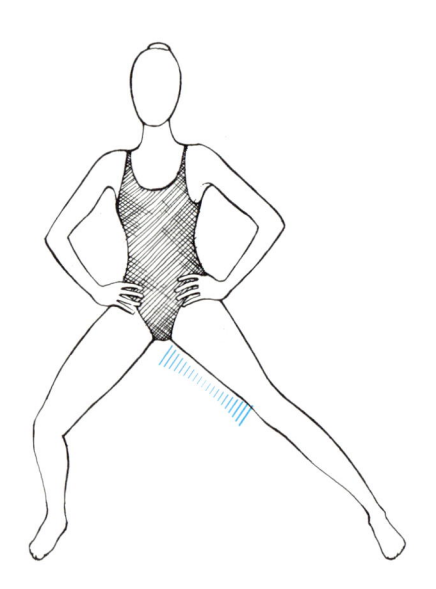

2 Adductor Stretch
Stretches inner thigh muscles.
Stand with legs wide apart and toes pointing forwards. Keep hands on hips, trunk upright. Drop right knee to carry weight until you feel stretch in left thigh. Hold, then repeat with other knee. Don't bounce or lean forwards or backwards.

3 Calf Stretch
Stretches calf muscles.
Lean against wall at 45° angle with arms out straight. Keep back straight, don't arch or lean your head back. Keep heels firmly on floor. Press hips forward until you feel a pull in your lower legs.

STARTING TO EXERCISE

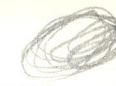

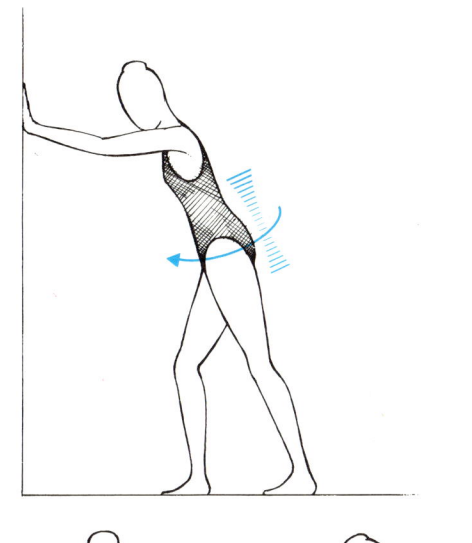

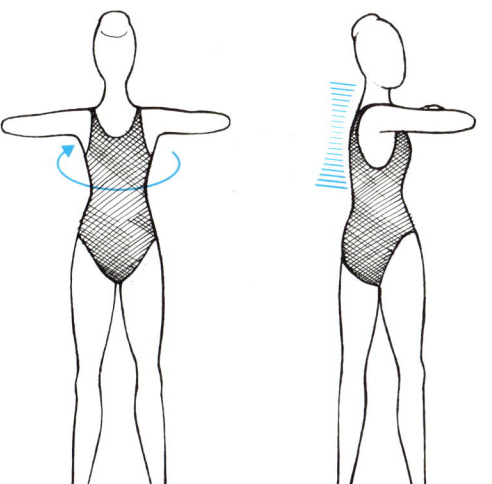

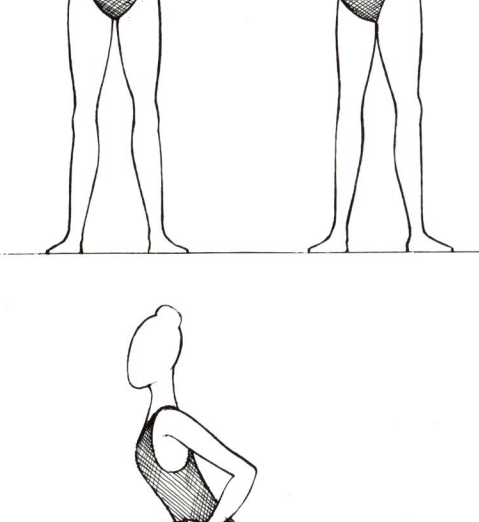

4 Hip Flexors
Stretches hips, calves and quads.
With hands on hips, move into a deep lunge position with front thigh straight and both feet pointing forwards. Drop weight towards bent front leg but keep trunk upright. Feel stretch and hold. Repeat with other leg.

5 Trunk Rotation
Increases hip, upper body, and back mobility.
Stand with feet hip-width apart and clasp fingers at shoulder level in front of chest, with elbows pointing out sideways. Keeping feet fixed forwards, turn head and whole body to side as far as possible and press into turn. Hold and repeat to other side.

6 Hip Rotation
Increases hip and lower back mobility and stretches calves.
Adopt same starting position as for calf stretch (3), but place right leg forward, bent at knee. Slowly rotate hip of left (rear) leg inwards. Hold. Change leg positions and repeat for other hip.

45

STARTING TO EXERCISE

Plan 1 15-25 years (8 weeks) (for exercise during pregnancy see pages 69-72)

Weeks	DAILY PATTER	DAILY STRETCH	DAY 1 WALK/JOG	DAY 2 SWIM/DANCE	DAY 3	DAY 4	DAY 5 CYCLE/SWIM	DAY 6 WALK/JOG	DAY 7
1	30 secs slow 15 secs fast 30 secs slow	Hold 5 secs Repeat 4 times	5 mins	10 mins	OFF	OFF	15 mins	5 mins	OFF
2	30 secs slow 15 secs fast 30 secs slow	Hold 5 secs Repeat 4 times	10 mins	15 mins	Except for Pattering and All Stretches	Except for Pattering and All Stretches	20 mins	10 mins	Except for Pattering and All Stretches
3	30 secs slow 30 secs fast 30 secs slow	Hold 5 secs Repeat 4 times	15 mins	20 mins	Except for Pattering and All Stretches	Except for Pattering and All Stretches	25 mins	15 mins	Except for Pattering and All Stretches
4	30 secs slow 30 secs fast 30 secs slow	Hold 10 secs Repeat 8 times	20 mins	25 mins	Except for Pattering and All Stretches	Except for Pattering and All Stretches	30 mins	20 mins	Except for Pattering and All Stretches
5	30 secs slow 45 secs fast 30 secs slow	Hold 10 secs Repeat 8 times	25 mins	30 mins	Except for Pattering and All Stretches	Except for Pattering and All Stretches	35 mins	25 mins	Except for Pattering and All Stretches
6	30 secs slow 45 secs fast 30 secs slow	Hold 10 secs Repeat 8 times	30 mins	35 mins	Except for Pattering and All Stretches	Except for Pattering and All Stretches	40 mins	30 mins	Except for Pattering and All Stretches
7	30 secs slow 60 secs fast 30 secs slow	Hold 10 secs Repeat 8 times	35 mins	40 mins	Except for Pattering and All Stretches	Except for Pattering and All Stretches	45 mins	35 mins	Except for Pattering and All Stretches
8	30 secs slow 60 secs fast 30 secs slow	Hold 10 secs Repeat 8 times	40 mins	45 mins	Except for Pattering and All Stretches	Except for Pattering and All Stretches	50 mins	40 mins	Except for Pattering and All Stretches

STARTING TO EXERCISE

Plan 2 25-35 years (12 weeks)
(for exercise during pregnancy see pages 69-72)

Weeks	DAILY PATTER	DAILY STRETCH	DAY 1 WALK/JOG	DAY 2 SWIM/DANCE	DAY 3	DAY 4	DAY 5 CYCLE/SWIM	DAY 6 WALK/JOG	DAY 7
1–2	20 secs 10 secs fast 20 secs slow	Hold 5 secs Repeat 4 times	5 mins	10 mins	OFF	OFF	15 mins	5 mins	OFF
3–4	20 secs slow 10 secs fast 20 secs slow	Hold 5 secs Repeat 4 times	10 mins	15 mins	Except for Pattering and All Stretches	Except for Pattering and All Stretches	20 mins	10 mins	Except for Pattering and All Stretches
5–6	30 secs slow 15 secs fast 30 secs slow	Hold 10 secs Repeat 4 times	15 mins	20 mins	Except for Pattering and All Stretches	Except for Pattering and All Stretches	25 mins	15 mins	Except for Pattering and All Stretches
7–8	30 secs slow 15 secs fast 30 secs slow	Hold 10 secs Repeat 4 times	20 mins	25 mins	Except for Pattering and All Stretches	Except for Pattering and All Stretches	30 mins	20 mins	Except for Pattering and All Stretches
9–10	30 secs slow 30 secs fast 30 secs slow	Hold 10 secs Repeat 8 times	25 mins	30 mins	Except for Pattering and All Stretches	Except for Pattering and All Stretches	35 mins	25 mins	Except for Pattering and All Stretches
11–12	30 secs slow 30 secs fast 30 secs slow	Hold 10 secs Repeat 8 times	30 mins	35 mins	Except for Pattering and All Stretches	Except for Pattering and All Stretches	40 mins	30 mins	Except for Pattering and All Stretches
13–14	30 secs slow 45 secs fast 30 secs slow	Hold 10 secs Repeat 8 times	35 mins	40 mins	Except for Pattering and All Stretches	Except for Pattering and All Stretches	45 mins	35 mins	Except for Pattering and All Stretches
15–16	30 secs slow 60 secs fast 30 secs slow	Hold 10 secs Repeat 8 times	40 mins	45 mins	Except for Pattering and All Stretches	Except for Pattering and All Stretches	50 mins	40 mins	Except for Pattering and All Stretches

STARTING TO EXERCISE

Plan 3 35-50 years (24 weeks)

(for exercise during pregnancy see pages 69-72)

Weeks	DAILY PATTER	DAILY STRETCH	DAY 1 WALK/JOG	DAY 2 SWIM/DANCE	DAY 3	DAY 4	DAY 5 CYCLE/SWIM	DAY 6 WALK/JOG	DAY 7
1–3	15 secs slow 10 secs fast 15 secs slow	Hold 5 secs Repeat 4 times	5 mins	10 mins	Except for Pattering and All Stretches	OFF	15 mins	5 mins	OFF
4–6	20 secs slow 10 secs fast 20 secs slow	Hold 10 secs Repeat 4 times	10 mins	15 mins	Except for Pattering and All Stretches	Except for Pattering and All Stretches	20 mins	10 mins	Except for Pattering and All Stretches
7–9	30 secs slow 15 secs fast 30 secs slow	Hold 10 secs Repeat 4 times	15 mins	20 mins	Except for Pattering and All Stretches	Except for Pattering and All Stretches	25 mins	15 mins	Except for Pattering and All Stretches
10–12	30 secs slow 15 secs fast 30 secs slow	Hold 10 secs Repeat 8 times	20 mins	25 mins	Except for Pattering and All Stretches	Except for Pattering and All Stretches	30 mins	20 mins	Except for Pattering and All Stretches
13–15	30 secs slow 30 secs fast 30 secs slow	Hold 10 secs Repeat 8 times	25 mins	30 mins	Except for Pattering and All Stretches	Except for Pattering and All Stretches	35 mins	25 mins	Except for Pattering and All Stretches
16–18	30 secs slow 30 secs fast 30 secs slow	Hold 10 secs Repeat 8 times	30 mins	35 mins	Except for Pattering and All Stretches	Except for Pattering and All Stretches	40 mins	30 mins	Except for Pattering and All Stretches
19–21	30 secs slow 45 secs fast 30 secs slow	Hold 10 secs Repeat 8 times	35 mins	40 mins	Except for Pattering and All Stretches	Except for Pattering and All Stretches	45 mins	35 mins	Except for Pattering and All Stretches
22–24	30 secs slow 60 secs fast 30 secs slow	Hold 10 secs Repeat 8 times	40 mins	45 mins	Except for Pattering and All Stretches	Except for Pattering and All Stretches	50 mins	40 mins	Except for Pattering and All Stretches

STARTING TO EXERCISE

Plan 4 50+ years (32 weeks)

Weeks	DAILY PATTER	DAILY STRETCH	DAY 1 WALK/JOG	DAY 2 SWIM/DANCE	DAY 3	DAY 4	DAY 5 CYCLE/SWIM	DAY 6 WALK/JOG	DAY 7
1–4	5 secs slow 5 secs fast 5 secs slow	Hold 5 secs Repeat 4 times	5 mins	10 mins	OFF	Except for Pattering and All Stretches	15 mins	5 mins	Except for Pattering and All Stretches
5–8	5 secs slow 10 secs fast 5 secs slow	Hold 5 secs Repeat 4 times	10 mins	15 mins	Except for Pattering and All Stretches	Except for Pattering and All Stretches	20 mins	10 mins	Except for Pattering and All Stretches
9–12	10 secs slow 10 secs fast 10 secs slow	Hold 10 secs Repeat 4 times	15 mins	20 mins	Except for Pattering and All Stretches	Except for Pattering and All Stretches	25 mins	15 mins	Except for Pattering and All Stretches
13–16	20 secs slow 10 secs fast 20 secs slow	Hold 10 secs Repeat 4 times	20 mins	25 mins	Except for Pattering and All Stretches	Except for Pattering and All Stretches	30 mins	20 mins	Except for Pattering and All Stretches
17–20	30 secs slow 15 secs fast 30 secs slow	Hold 10 secs Repeat 8 times	25 mins	30 mins	Except for Pattering and All Stretches	Except for Pattering and All Stretches	35 mins	25 mins	Except for Pattering and All Stretches
21–24	30 secs slow 30 secs fast 30 secs slow	Hold 10 secs Repeat 8 times	30 mins	35 mins	Except for Pattering and All Stretches	Except for Pattering and All Stretches	40 mins	30 mins	Except for Pattering and All Stretches
25–28	30 secs slow 45 secs fast 30 secs slow	Hold 10 secs Repeat 8 times	35 mins	40 mins	Except for Pattering and All Stretches	Except for Pattering and All Stretches	45 mins	35 mins	Except for Pattering and All Stretches
29–32	30 secs slow 60 secs fast 30 secs slow	Hold 10 secs Repeat 8 times	40 mins	45 mins	Except for Pattering and All Stretches	Except for Pattering and All Stretches	50 mins	40 mins	Except for Pattering and All Stretches

Sickness and Injury

When Not to Exercise

>If you have a temperature
>If you have a cold
>If you have 'flu

Participating in sport at these times could have serious side effects and can make the illness last longer. Since they are all likely to settle within a few days it is best to take a short break. Occasionally after a bad dose of 'flu you may feel tired and lethargic for some weeks. If this happens then strenuous exercise should be avoided until you feel able to tackle it. However once the feverish time has passed you can begin gentle stretching and some walking so that you don't lose your fitness altogether.

Fatigue

Exercise will make you tired, more so when you are starting up. You need to learn the difference between 'healthy' tiredness and fatigue resulting from overdoing it. Generally speaking, 'healthy' tiredness is only felt after exercise and is usually followed by a 'good night's sleep' with complete recovery by the next day. If you have overdone things you are likely to feel tired before exercising and the activity will take a lot of effort with consequent diminution in enjoyment. Sleep is unlikely to make you feel refreshed.

When this happens either take a break or temporarily switch to an alternative, less exacting sport. In the long run this is far better than pushing on through fatigue with risk of injury. This type of tiredness must be distinguished from laziness. On a cold, dark, winter's morning or a wet foggy evening, few of us feel like getting up and going out no matter how much we enjoy the planned activity. In this instance once up and out and enjoying ourselves in our chosen sport then that 'lazy tiredness' is forgotten.

Prevention of Injury

Although some injuries cannot be prevented, many can be by attention to a few simple principles.

Warming up: Before beginning any exercise or sport a period should be spent warming up. This has the effect of increasing muscle blood flow so that muscles are 'prepared' for more strenuous activity. The muscle temperature increases with the result that muscle contraction is facilitated. Gentle running on the spot or a slowed down version of the planned activity for a few minutes will suffice. In addition, some stretching of the muscles to be used should be undertaken. This has the effect of preparing the muscles for both the repetitive muscle contraction of the planned exercise as well as for sudden unexpected stretch that may occur.

Training: A *gradual* increase of the chosen sport is important in preventing overuse injuries. Too much too quickly is likely to cause tissue breakdown. Pain is the body's warning sign and should be an alert to ease off. Pushing through pain can damage the affected part. Such pain is to be distinguished from the aching of tired muscles which is eased by rest, stretching, a warm bath or massage.

Technique: Doing a sport badly can result in injury. This is particularly so in racket sports and throwing events—eg, javelin. So when learning a new sport get expert advice to learn how to do it correctly and avoid injury.

Equipment: The wrong equipment can result in injury. A racket that is too heavy or with the wrong-sized grip results in strain of the muscles involved in holding the racket. The wrong shoes may cause injury by having inadequate shock absorption, excessive or inadequate grip of the sole. Where protective equipment is needed, such as a hat for riding, be sure to use it to reduce the severity of injury if you are unfortunate enough to have an accident.

Environment: This applies to both the surfaces on which exercise is undertaken and the prevailing climatic conditions. Exercise undertaken on one surface cannot be immediately transferred to another without risk of

STARTING TO EXERCISE

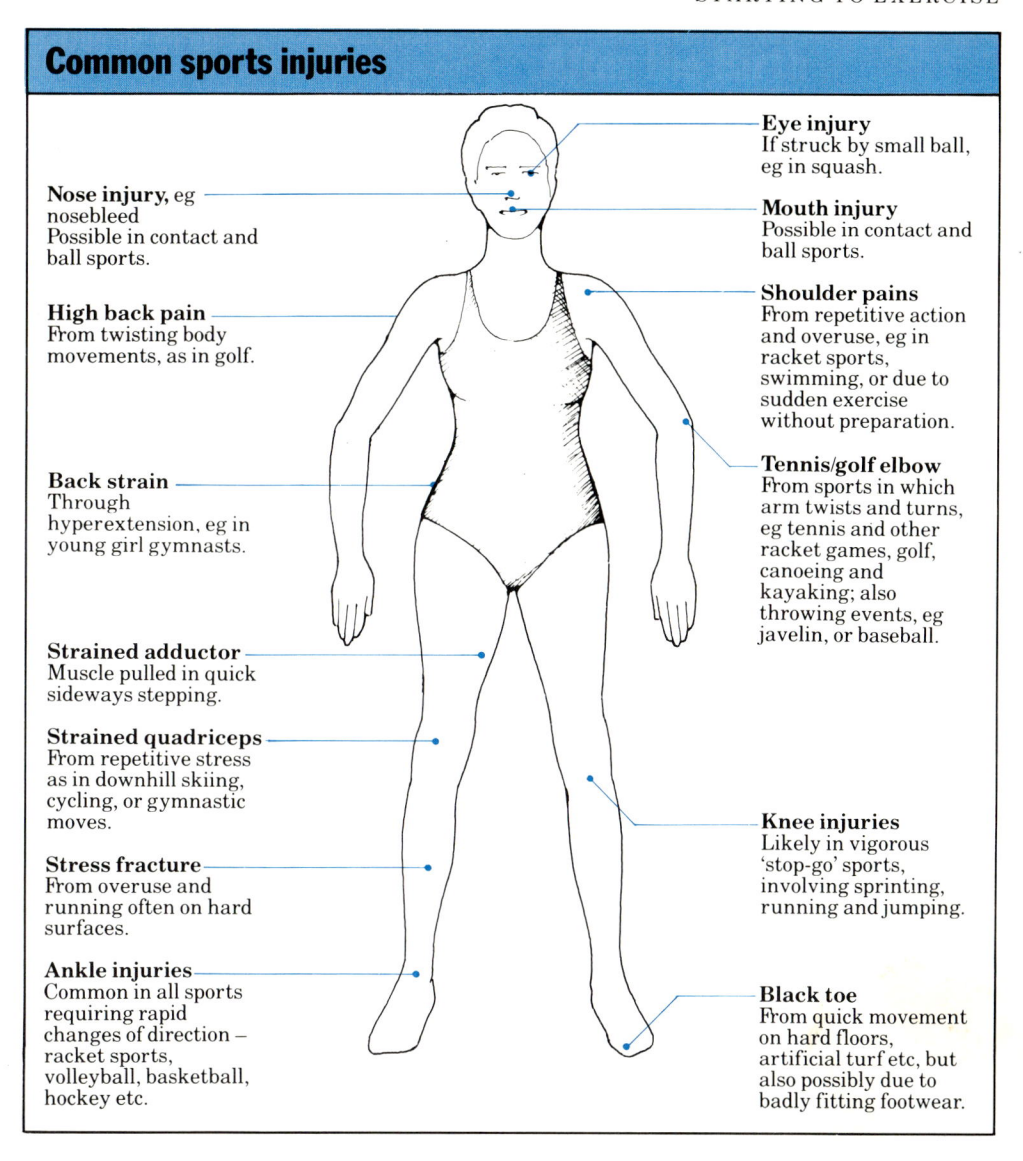

Common sports injuries

Eye injury
If struck by small ball, eg in squash.

Nose injury, eg nosebleed
Possible in contact and ball sports.

Mouth injury
Possible in contact and ball sports.

Shoulder pains
From repetitive action and overuse, eg in racket sports, swimming, or due to sudden exercise without preparation.

High back pain
From twisting body movements, as in golf.

Back strain
Through hyperextension, eg in young girl gymnasts.

Tennis/golf elbow
From sports in which arm twists and turns, eg tennis and other racket games, golf, canoeing and kayaking; also throwing events, eg javelin, or baseball.

Strained adductor
Muscle pulled in quick sideways stepping.

Strained quadriceps
From repetitive stress as in downhill skiing, cycling, or gymnastic moves.

Knee injuries
Likely in vigorous 'stop-go' sports, involving sprinting, running and jumping.

Stress fracture
From overuse and running often on hard surfaces.

Ankle injuries
Common in all sports requiring rapid changes of direction – racket sports, volleyball, basketball, hockey etc.

Black toe
From quick movement on hard floors, artificial turf etc, but also possibly due to badly fitting footwear.

injury. For example, hockey on grass is different from hockey played on a hard pitch or artificial turf, and training on the intended surface should obviously precede competition on that surface. Running on a cambered road, always in the same direction can result in injury as it has the effect of producing an apparent inequality of leg length, stressing the downward or 'longer' leg.

In hot conditions it is important to wear light coloured clothes of natural materials, and to drink plenty of fluids to avoid heat injury. In cold conditions warm clothing is vital and a good warm-up becomes even more important. High winds and rain can exacerbate cold exposure so suitable clothing should be worn, or carried, in environments where sudden weather changes can occur—eg, when cross-country skiing or hill walking.

Body structure: Certain individuals, because of their build, are unsuited to certain activities since they may be more susceptible to injury. For example, if you are slightly knock-kneed or bowlegged you should avoid activities with repetitive stress on the

51

STARTING TO EXERCISE

knees such as running. If you have excessive movements in the joints, contact sports and the martial arts should be avoided as you are more at risk of injury when force is applied to the joints.

Acute Injuries
I.C.E.
Ice—Compression—Elevation—is a useful motto for a wide variety of soft tissue injuries ranging from sprained ankles to muscle tears or 'pulls'. As soon as possible after injury, apply ice or other cold substance—eg, a pack of frozen peas, or cold water—to the injured part—whether muscle or joint. This will reduce bleeding into the damaged tissues if applied for 15–20 minutes, but take care to avoid an ice burn by wrapping the ice in a damp towel and using baby oil on the skin first. Repeat this three or four times during the first 48 hours. Ice also reduces the pain although in the first few minutes the cooling is itself painful. Where practicable a compressive bandage should be applied to minimise the swelling, followed by elevation of the injured part to enhance drainage. The bandage should provide comfortable support without being too tight.

After the first few days, if there is still pain and swelling, then contrast bathing is a useful method to encourage reduction of swelling. This consists of alternate applications of hot and cold using 1 minute of heat—eg, a hot water bottle—followed by 2 minutes of ice, this being repeated four or five times in succession and undertaken two or three times a day.

Pain may well be a deciding factor in considering when to start exercising after injury. If you cannot do your chosen sport try another that you can manage. If you have injured your leg, for example, try swimming—using arms only if necessary to maintain cardiovascular fitness. If the arm is injured try cycling providing you can balance.

Prolonged and recurrent injury often result from a persistent weakness in the tissues which has developed after the original injury. Although the tissues damaged may have healed, a weakness which is secondary to the original

Ice
Wrap icepack in cloth (to prevent ice burn, or use cold water if no ice available) and apply to injured area for 20 minutes. Do this 4 times a day for two days. This reduces bleeding from torn blood vessels.

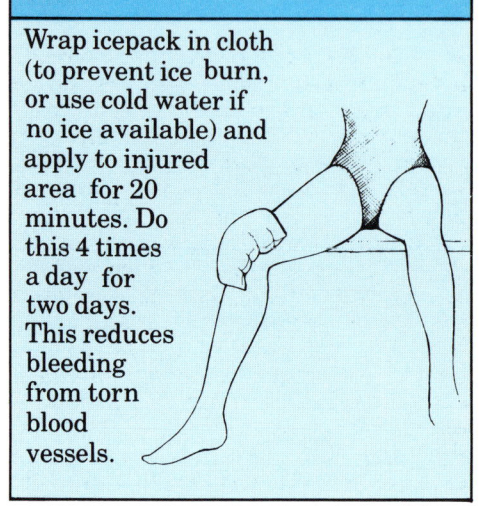

Compression
Between icings, bandage area firmly (but not so tightly that it is uncomfortable) in order to contain swelling.

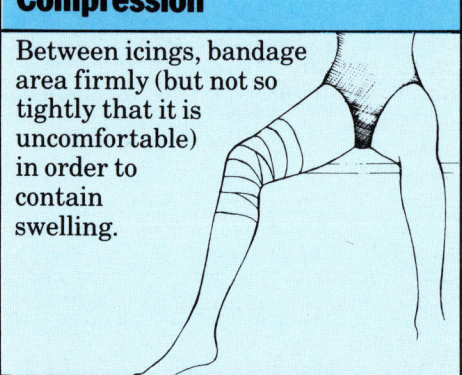

Elevation
Elevate injured area as often as possible and for as long as possible. Allows blood to flow back to the heart and reduces pressure of fluid.

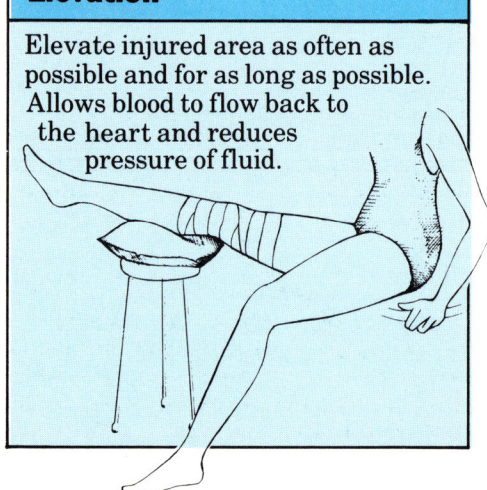

injury can produce continuation of symptoms and predispose to further injury.

Muscle injuries: These usually result in tearing of some muscle fibres and the number of fibres torn will determine the severity of the injury. In addition to actual muscle damage, some blood vessels are damaged which produces bleeding into the muscle. I.C.E. is used to minimise this. The damaged area in the muscle heals by the formation of scar tissue, but this does not stretch in the same way as the muscle. It is therefore important after the first 48 hours (or longer if there has been extensive muscle injury) to *gradually* apply a stretch to the affected muscle so that the scar tissue is made more extensible and does not limit the subsequent *mobility*. The aim should be to obtain the same flexibility on the injured side as on the non-injured side. Initially there will be a tightness at the injury site, but if the area is stretched regularly this will disappear. It is important to apply a controlled stretch and not a 'bouncing stretch'.

The other factor to regain following muscle injury is *strength*. This will return, to some extent, with use, but if there is considerable damage then more specfic strengthening will be required, with exercises utilising body weight as resistance or using weights, the exercises depending on the site of the injury. It is failure to regain *mobility* and *strength* which can result in recurrence of injury or prolonged symptoms. Muscle injuries can be reduced by paying attention to warm up and doing regular mobility exercises. As for the healing time of torn muscle, if the bleeding that occurs is between the bundles of muscle fibres (intermuscular haematoma) then it can drain outwards and all may be well after about 10 days. If the bleeding is within the muscle (intramuscular haematoma) it cannot easily be dispersed and the length of disability will be about three weeks.

Ankle sprain: This is over-stretching of the ankle ligaments and one of the most common sporting injuries. Use I.C.E. in the first 48 hours. Follow this with activities to restore *mobility*,

STARTING TO EXERCISE

strength, and *balance*, which need to be worked at gradually within the limits of pain. Mobility, as in the case of muscle injuries, should eventually be the same as that in the unaffected ankle. In some instances mobility will be increased due to excessive stretching of the ligaments and then *strength* becomes of paramount importance in order to try to compensate for and to control excessive ankle movement. Again strengthening can be done using body weight or actual weights. Recurrent ankle injuries are often caused by failure to attend to balance. Problems with balance result from damage to the nerves supplying the joint. The ideal way of re-educating the balance mechanisms is with a specially designed 'wobble board'. A simple, but effective, alternative is to practise balancing on the floor, standing only on the injured ankle. When this is possible for several minutes at a time, it should then be done with the eyes closed.

Following an injury it is important to return *gradually* to activities, as over-enthusiasm may result in re-injury. One danger of returning to sport too early is the risk of developing secondary injuries either as a result of weakness putting extra strain on previously unaffected parts or due to picking up an abnormal technique as a result of the injury. When injured, maintain hard-earned fitness by doing other activities. Swimming is an ideal exercise in the case of leg injuries as it avoids weight bearing. Cycling is a good way to maintain cardiovascular fitness even if an arm is injured.

Chronic Injuries

These usually result from overuse, and they will not go away without modifying your exercise pattern. Try to establish why you have developed the injury in order to avoid another in the future. Switch to another sport which avoids stressing the injured part, which may take several months to recover, especially if it has already been present for several months. Short term pain relief may be obtained by massaging the injured area with an ice cube. If the injury is not improving despite relative rest seek advice from a chartered physiotherapist or a doctor.

Major Body Changes

Women undergo many body changes during their lives — most quite major. How a woman copes with these changes, and the bearing they have on the quality of her life, can be greatly assisted with the help of sport and exercise. In this chapter, we look at puberty, menstruation and contraception, pregnancy, the menopause, and growing older, and highlight the contribution exercise can make in every instance.

Puberty

This is the gradual development of physical, sexual maturity. It takes place over several years and culminates with the onset of menstruation (menarche). From about 8 years, increasing levels of hormones produced by the pituitary gland in the brain allow the ovaries to respond to the primary female sex hormone, oestrogen. At first these changes are heralded by a rapid increase in growth rate—such that girls are often considerably taller than their male contemporaries; but there then follows the development of the secondary sex characteristics.

Internally, the Fallopian tubes, uterus and vagina all increase in size, while externally, there is enlargement of the labia and clitoris and gradual breast development (influenced also by progesterone). Later pubic hair appears (due to other hormones) and then hair in the armpits (axillae). The appearance of these secondary sex characteristics may be as early as 8 years or as late as 17, but the average is around 12 years. It has become younger with successive generations, probably owing to better nutrition.

Puberty is undoubtedly a time of major body change. Regrettably, perhaps, there is no cultural or social recognition of this incipient womanhood and so we tend not to take adolescents seriously. Presumably, this is because psychological and emotional maturity—the components which make for adulthood—have yet to evolve, and yet such an attitude only serves to exacerbate any emotional conflict and inhibit the natural assertion of newly-acquired identity. Nevertheless, puberty can be a time of wonderment and pride holding many secret delights: the gradually evolving sexual body, the first indication of fertility, perhaps even the first bra, are all worthy of celebration.

At some point, sex will be confronted, deliberately or not. It is important that a young woman has all the facts before her, knows about contraception and is disabused of myths surrounding virginity and the hymen, and the notion that sex, and later marriage, is all.

Why Exercise in Puberty

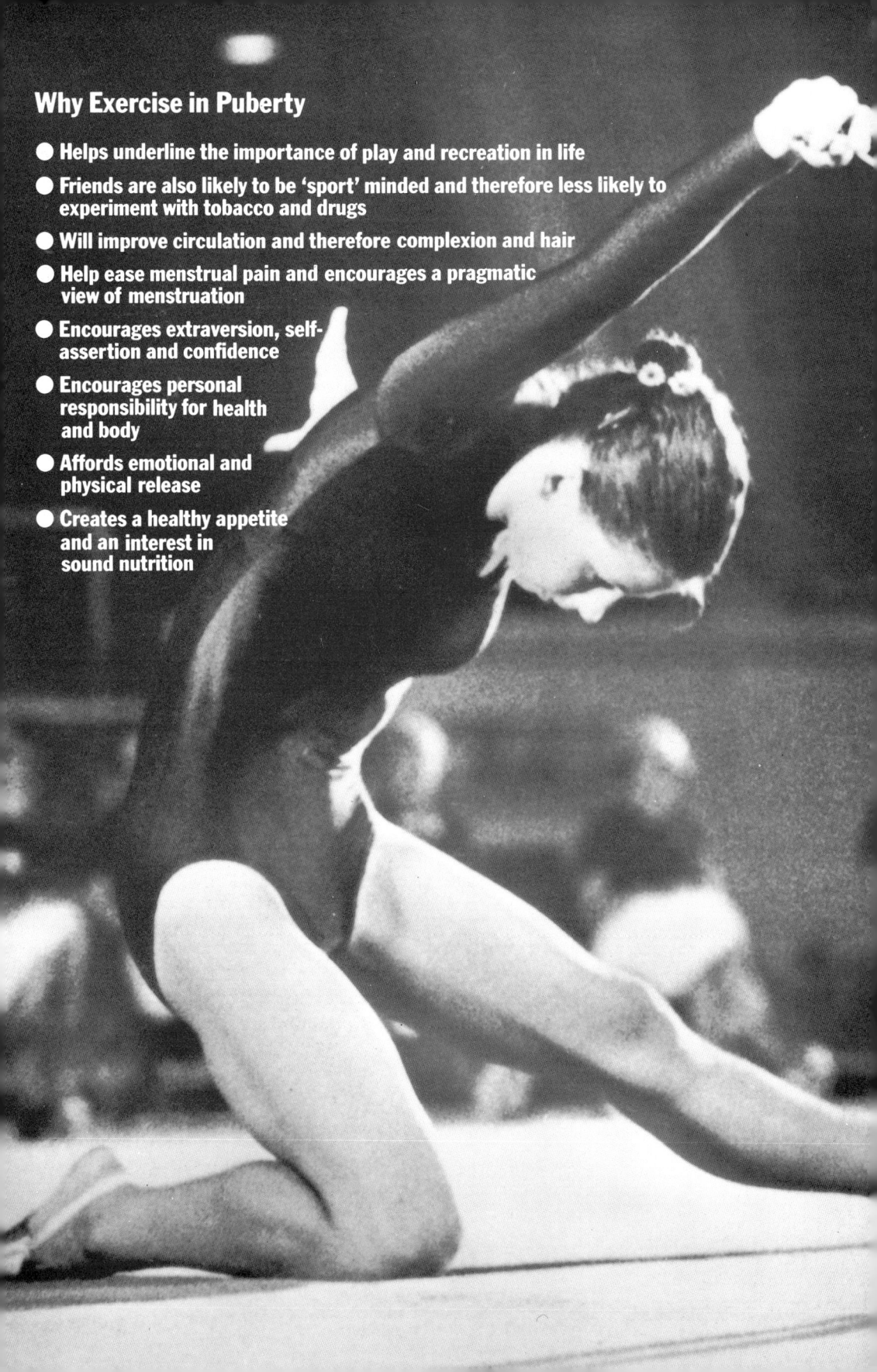

- Helps underline the importance of play and recreation in life
- Friends are also likely to be 'sport' minded and therefore less likely to experiment with tobacco and drugs
- Will improve circulation and therefore complexion and hair
- Help ease menstrual pain and encourages a pragmatic view of menstruation
- Encourages extraversion, self-assertion and confidence
- Encourages personal responsibility for health and body
- Affords emotional and physical release
- Creates a healthy appetite and an interest in sound nutrition

MAJOR BODY CHANGES

Many girls have casual sex at this age in order to off-load their virginity and prove themselves. These are rarely happy experiences and may only serve to reduce the sense of self-worth.

Menarche
This is the first period. It is a date that most women remember and also marks the point at which daughters endeavour to separate themselves from their mothers asserting their identities as women and in their own right.

The first period is usually a great

MAJOR BODY CHANGES

surprise, even though it has been expected for some time. It is usually greeted quite emotionally, and while some girls may be thrilled by this sign of womanhood, others may feel ashamed or embarrassed, or simply that they are not yet ready.

During the preceding months, there is usually a creamy, white vaginal discharge as a result of the increased levels of oestrogen. This is natural and healthy. The period itself may be obviously bloody or thick and brownish; it may last 24 hours or 10 days and be very slight or very heavy. The first few periods are usually irregular and anovulatory—ie, no eggs are produced.

Tampons or Pads: The choice is yours. While pads may satisfy a certain curiosity in that the evidence of bleeding is visible, they can be bulky and also chafe the legs. Because they are worn externally, there may be fears that they can be seen, might drop out or be smelly. This last should not be a problem if the pads are changed 3–4 times a day and before going to bed.

Tampons create none of these problems. They are extremely convenient, totally unobtrusive, they can slip into a purse or pocket, can be worn while swimming, having a bath, riding a horse or bicycle, and they *can* be worn by young girls. If you want to try tampons, try the slimmest size first, and often the ones with applicators are the easiest to use initially. Don't buy scented ones (or pads for that matter) which can encourage infection.

Read the instructions, take a look at yourself and relax (after a bath is a good time). Be gentle. If you have any difficulty inserting the tampon, relax, rub some KY jelly around it and try again. Don't use petroleum jelly, which is not water-soluble. If it still won't go in, forget about it, use a pad and try another time. You should not be able to feel the tampon inside you. If you can, or it hurts when you sit down or bend, it means the tampon is not in far enough and has been 'trapped' by your external vaginal muscles; pull it out and try again.

Tampons should be changed at least as often as pads, and remember to take the last one out at the end of period.

Diet: What you eat can affect how you feel (and look) during a period. Because you will probably be bleeding every month, you will also be losing iron—an important component of blood—and you could become anaemic. One way to avoid this is to eat iron-rich foods—liver, eggs, wholegrain cereals and dark green vegetables—and increase your intake of vitamin C. Calcium-rich foods (cheese, milk, sardines, yoghurt) may help with cramps, while wholefoods, because they are digested slowly, can help with feelings of faintness and also with constipation. If you're thirsty, drink water or fruit juice rather than milk. Milk is a very concentrated food and doesn't really quench your thirst. It also contains a lot of calories and could cause you to put on weight unnecessarily if you drink a lot.

Weight

Puberty is accompanied by an increase in body weight as oestrogen lays down additional body fat around the buttocks, hips and breasts. The number of fat cells that we have at puberty are what we have for life. 'Puppy fat' is a term used to cover a multitude of sins, and similarly, 'glands' are rarely the problem that many mothers make out. While there may be a familial tendency to overweight, the causes are less genetic than simply following bad eating habits and eating too much. So, however much we slim, diet, lose weight later in life, the fat cells are still there, even if they have shrunk.

Exercise, whether it's in the form of sport or 'Keep Fit', is a pleasurable and painless way to work off excess calories. Britain's Health Education Council points out that 'most overweight children are unhappy about their futures, although they may not show it'.

Setting the Pattern

There is no reason why exercise cannot be commenced for the first time during puberty even if a girl has led a relatively sedentary life previously. By encouraging regular exercise during puberty, the pattern of a lifestyle with physical recreation as one part of it is more likely to be established for the remainder of the adult life. As it is sometimes an occasion when sport is discontinued on account of embarrassment, efforts should be made to overcome this stressing the advantages of regular exercise—perhaps the most attractive at this age being the control of body weight and social opportunities that it provides.

Before puberty, many girls see sport as fun and exciting but unfortunately, once the first period arrives become distracted by other things and forget all about the pleasure—and benefits—of sport and exercise. In Britain, where figures are higher than in the USA, only one girl in three plays sport after leaving school.

Muscle Bound: One fear that girls sometimes have about taking sport at all seriously is of developing bulging muscles. The fact is that it is very difficult for a woman to build up her muscles, however hard she works at it. At the same time, she *can* increase the *strength* of her muscles. Research by Dr J H Wilmore found that a concentrated ten-week training programme for non-

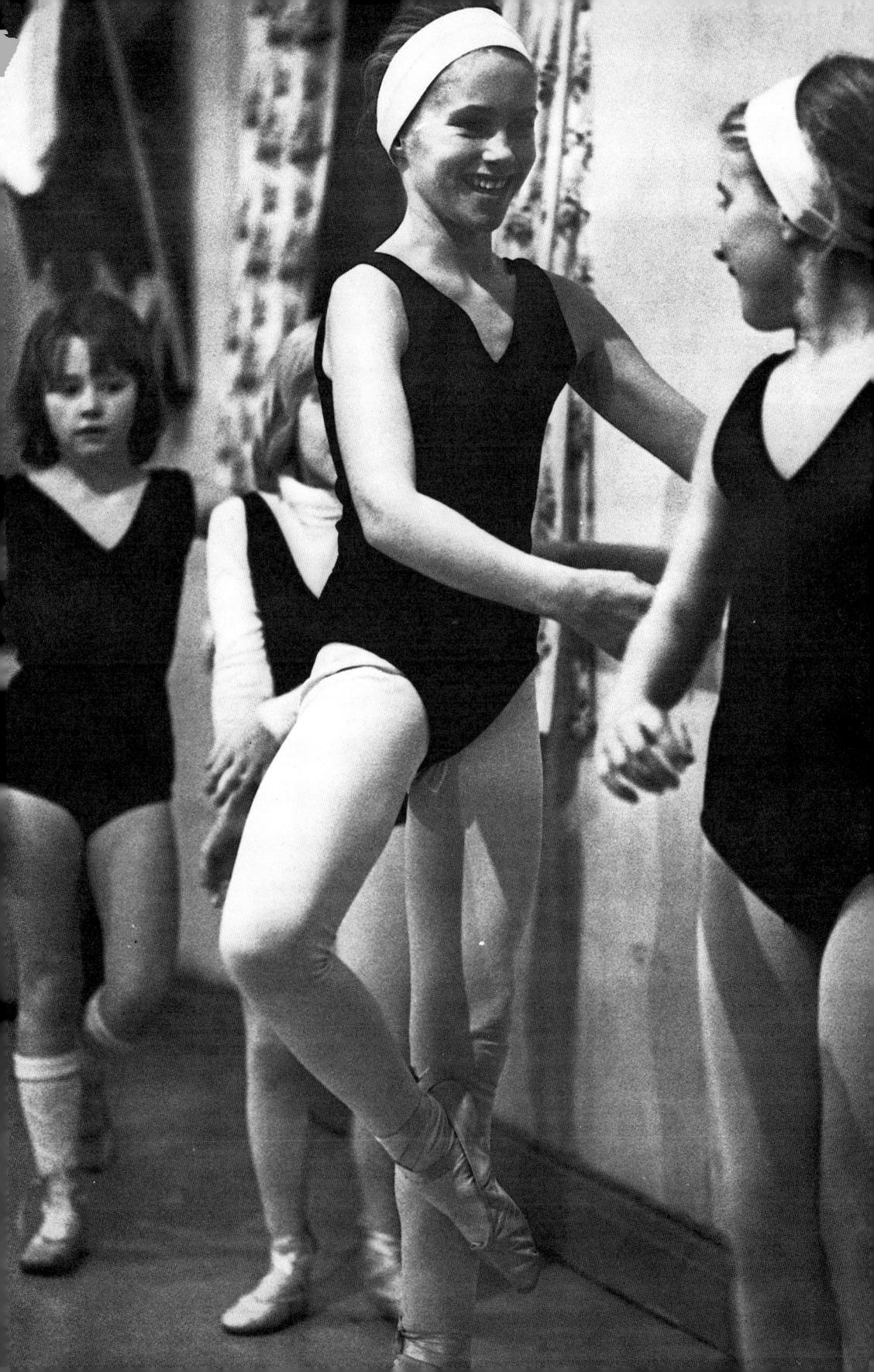

athletic girls increased their muscular strength 30% with little increase in the size of the muscles.

What Sort of Exercise?

Deep into the teens, boys' hearts and lungs tend to be about 25% bigger than girls', but medical experts realise that this is another example of tradition rather than genetics. This is the age when aerobic exercise is most effective, and we are now seeing that women who have taken part in aerobic (stamina-building) events like running, swimming, cycling and cross-country skiing can develop tremendous ability to convert oxygen intake into energy. Joan Benoit, for example, winner of the 1984 Olympic marathon, has a more efficient heart/lung system than some male athletes of comparable calibre.

Just as schools emphasise an all-round education until the mid-teens at the earliest, so sport and exercise should offer a wide range of choice. Few sports provide all-round fitness, so a girl who plays nothing but tennis could end up doing little anaerobic (sprint or speed) work, and would rely on exercising one half of her growing body (on the racket side) to the exclusion of the other. By limiting a girl to one sport, greater ability in a totally different sport may remain undiscovered, and she may even suffer socially by alienating herself from friends.

On the other hand, properly monitored, girls should not have their sporting ambitions stifled. In 1984, the first girl ever to play in the Little League Baseball World Series came from Belgium, 12-year-old Victoria Roche, a reserve outfielder. Girls have played Little League baseball since 1974, when the sport itself recognised that girls were as able as boys.

Training: Hard anaerobic work should be avoided until two years after the final growth spurt which can occur at any time between 10 and 18 years. Certainly no training involving weights or similar stresses should be used until the age of 18. Athletics coach Ken Seddington who looks after Olympic competitors spelt it out in *Sport and Leisure* magazine: 'It's all too easy to push a young athlete too far. The process of *growing* takes an enormous toll of the human body and if a youngster trains too hard, either growth is affected or (s)he is just *too tired to benefit.*'

The same is true of hard aerobic training. He goes on to say, 'The tendons in particular are stretched to the limit by the teenager's rapid growth. Over-enthusiastic training can lead to damage and scar-tissue which will be a problem for the rest of the career. Over-enthusiastic training is more likely to make a youngster leave sport than love it, either through the frustration of being side-lined by injury, or through fear of the pain.'

Too Much Exercise?

In America, physicians have long ago spotted what they call 'socially approved athletic child abuse'. In Britain, too, physiotherapists are seeing more and more 'battered child athletes'. The fault lies totally at the door of parents and ill-informed coaches who try to live out their own sporting fantasies through their children or who are influenced by the success of young gymnasts, swimmers and tennis players who star on TV screens round the world.

Bones: Children's bones are quite soft, and do not stop growing until the late teens. In fact, each bone is made up of separate parts (ends and middle) that are slowly fusing together. Too much stress and strain on these bones could retard the fusion for as much as two years, and even cause deformity. Common injury spots are the heel, just below the knee, and the base of the spine. In the past these pains were mis-labelled as 'diseases', but they are really the effect of overuse and overloading. Sever's disease (heel), Osgood-Schlatter's disease (shin) and spondylolysis (lower back) should all be rested properly under medical supervision.

Muscles: As mentioned, children grow in spurts, so they are particularly vulnerable to injury during one of these growth periods. The body also tires more quickly and muscles are more prone to strains.

Joints: For many sports medicine experts, the joints are the most worrying part of the athletic child's anatomy. As the emergence of young sports stars is so recent, there has not been time to build up a picture of the long-term effect of stress and strain on joints.

Psychology: The damage to these young athletes is not only physical. Top class athletes know that the way to build up to a marathon is by running *short* events. The official minimum age for competition in marathons is 18 and until that age many top-class runners have not competed over distances greater than 6 miles (10 km). A child will never improve her time by running long distances, and the psychological depression of competing without improving usually leads to the abandoning of sport and exercise altogether.

Sports Injuries in Children

British Olympic team doctor, Malcolm Read is always especially suspicious about children who are brought to him with sporting injuries. 'You see most girls pushed in gymnastics. Certainly in Britain I spend so much time having to hold back parents, while I try to find out what the girl actually wants to do. Girls often claim that they're injured in order to get out of doing the sport because they're being pressured. If there is no injury, then I have to concentrate on the parents to persuade them that they're overdoing it.'

If the injuries are genuine, then very special attention has to be taken, especially if they are of the type that can cause problems in later life.

Menstruation

In many societies, menstruation has always been shrouded in myth, magic and taboo. The mysterious bloody emission—which of itself is nothing more than waste tissue—is a potent indicator of fertility, a most valued and irreducible life-force. Because this natural 28-day life-cycle coincided with the waxing and waning of the moon, women who were menstruating were regarded as witches or portents of evil-doing, and while we may think we are far removed from such cultures, many superstitions about menstruation still prevail.

How a woman reacts to the monthly shedding of the lining of her uterus is as much influenced by her early conditioning and expectation as by her own personality, beliefs, health and

Anorexia Nervosa

This is a serious psychological illness which affects mainly (though by no means exclusively) adolescent girls. The mortality rate is high (up to 10%) and treatment lies in medical intervention often with psychiatric support and counselling. The causes and maintaining factors are complex and may not be the same. The illness is often triggered by over-zealous dieting which then gets out of hand. Or, there may have been some physical or emotional trauma such as the menarche, death within the family or of a loved one, or a broken relationship. There is frequently a strong but frustrated desire for love and recognition. The thwarting of these emotions leads to intense avoidance behaviour and punitive starvation.

The role of sport and exercise in anorexia nervosa is problematic since hyperactivity is often already present and any pressure exerted on the anorexic to participate in sports may also make matters worse.

However, properly *supervised* exercise may well be beneficial by helping to untie the psychological knots which have led to the anorexia, and by gradually instilling a more rational sense of control and mastery over one's life and body.

Perhaps of more significance, is the role of sport and exercise in preventing anorexia and in preventing recurrent episodes, or the heavy smoking and drinking which is now seen to feature in women in their 20s and 30s who were anorexic in their teens.

lifestyle. The marketing of disposable sanitary wear may have liberated us from the ritual chore of washing bloody cloths, but still, menstruation is something some women would prefer to ignore. It is a 'curse' upon one half of the human race supposedly making us weaker and therefore not in total command of our faculties.

For some women, a period is the manifest sign of the end of one cycle and the beginning of another and brings with it a tremendous release of creative and sexual energy. For others it is a time of calm and 'cosiness'—and the first day in particular may bring about a wish for solitude and reflection—almost a withdrawing back into the womb. More obviously perhaps, a period signals the lack of a pregnancy which to many women brings great relief, though for others the bloody issue signifies loss.

The advent and widespread use of the Pill has done much to remove women from the intricate workings of their bodies. Undoubtedly it is favoured because of its effective control of pregnancy, but less positively, perhaps, its popularity also belies the fact that many women continue to feel at odds with their bodies and its reproductive idiosyncrasies.

However, because of better nutrition, causing an ever-earlier menarche, and social awareness about population control so that women are not having as many children, women in the 1980s are subject to more menstrual cycles and episodes of bleeding than their grandmothers ever were. It would be interesting and undoubtedly worthwhile to investigate the effect of these continuous cycles, month after month, on a woman's mental and physical health.

The Effect of Menstruation

The physiological effect of menstruation although it will vary from woman to woman and cycle to cycle, is probably universal. Its onset is usually heralded by premonitory signs such as low backache, nausea, forgetfulness, sensations of heaviness or 'pulling' in the vagina and there may be a heightened sense of awareness. Once the flow begins, the lassitude of the premenstrual days may give way to downright fatigue followed by a feeling of being drained as the flow becomes established. All of these feelings depend on many factors, but not least on the amount of blood lost and the general state of health. Although the average amount of blood lost may be less than a teacupful, it is the chronic loss of blood month after month which depletes iron stores and can lead to iron-deficiency anaemia and exacerbate fatigue.

A combination of adequate sleep, sound nutrition, and exercise can do much to counteract the effects of menstruation.

On Exercise: It is probably very difficult to evaluate the effect of periods on exercise at competition level since many sportswomen will have chosen the Pill for its blanket effect on the menstrual cycle. However, probably the majority will say that they perform less well during a period. This is possibly because they expect less of themselves, but also probably because they are genuinely fatigued and drained of certain essential minerals. Problems of balance and co-ordination are more likely to be premenstrual than to arise during the period itself.

Dysmenorrhoea (painful periods)

Many healthy women have some menstrual discomfort but only about 5% have sufficient pain to seek treatment and in about half of these, pain is enough to interrupt work. It usually begins soon after puberty and commonly ceases after child-bearing. There are many theories as to the cause of painful periods, but it is probably due to reduced blood supply to the uterus (womb) as it contracts strongly enough to shut off its own circulation. Psychological factors undoubtedly accentuate symptoms, especially in adolescents who are led to expect menstrual disability and in older girls there may be a fear of body abnormality. Thus it is very important before periods begin for mothers to adopt positive attitudes rather than to predict or accept that periods are going to be a problem. A well-prepared girl is less likely to be disabled by any new symptoms that she may develop.

Sex and Exercise

Sex is certainly physical exercise and as Dr William Masters pointed out in his report 'Human Sexual Reponses' back in 1966: 'A person who has a good physical fitness invariably functions more effectively sexually than a person in poor shape. Sexual function is a physiological process and every physiological process works better in a good state of health.' A heart rate of 180 beats per minute has been measured during intercourse, which is pretty high when you realise that top class athletes reach between 180 and 220 during competition! This leads to the reasonable theory that a physically fit person finds it easier to maintain the intensity which adds to the satisfaction of lovemaking. Having said that, all the puffing and panting might give the impression that we are exhausting ourselves, but a brisk walk rather than a five-mile walk is nearer the mark in terms of calories burned—150 calories! Nevertheless, sex *is* good for you: it is relaxing because research shows that after love making we fall asleep sooner, sleep more deeply and even considerably longer.

The only problem is that you might get fitter than your partner and then feel less than satisfied. A gentle explanation that this is due to exercise, outlining the benefits should persuade him to join you...

As mentioned, in general, athletic, professional and other active women seem to be less incapacitated by pain than their inactive sisters. It is uncertain whether the self-discipline and pain tolerance they have developed during training enables them to put up with more pain. They may have a natural resistance to pain or reduced perception of it, allowing them to be more active. Regardless of the exact mechanism, sport and exercise may have short- and long-term beneficial effects on pain for many women.

If the pain is severe, aspirin and other tablets—eg, ibuprofen, can be taken to counteract prostaglandins, natural substances in the body which are one factor related to pain. 600 mgs or 2 tablets of soluble aspirin can be taken with each meal, commencing either with the onset of pain or prior to it, if this begins on a known day of the cycle.

Amenorrhoea (absence of periods)

The commonest cause of this in women between 15 and 45 is pregnancy! There are, however, many other causes; one common and often unappreciated reason is stress. Thus, for young girls moving away from home, having examinations, or family pressures are all factors which may result in periods stopping. Exercise, though a positive form of stress, can also have this effect. Amenorrhoea is termed 'primary' when menstruation has never occurred—which may be due to late development or some structural or pathological cause—and 'secondary' when periods stop for reasons other than pregnancy. Amenorrhoea does not necessarily mean you are not ovulating—although it may be the case—but it certainly does mean that ovulation is not occurring regularly and, therefore, fertility is reduced. However, pregnancy may still occur and contraceptive cover is necessary. If any of a variety of stresses have produced the amenorrhoea, then removal or reduction in the stress results in a return to normal menstruation and regular ovulation. If amenorrhoea persists for longer than 6 months, then you should see your doctor.

Much publicity has been given to amenorrhoea in athletes. It may be that the stress of high level training is the factor, or this and a combination of reduced body weight as there is certainly a relationship between a fall in body weight and cessation of menstruation. Generally speaking, you need a minimum of 17% body fat for the menarche to occur at all, and a minimum of 20% body fat for menstruation to occur regularly.

MAJOR BODY CHANGES

Premenstrual Tension

PMT has probably always existed but for many reasons has taken a long time to be recognised. It is likely that all women at some point in their lives suffer or have suffered from PMT. The exact cause is unknown but several hormones have been named as culprits—oestrogen/progesterone imbalance, aldosterone, and an increase in prolactin levels. While there is no psychological or personality condition predisposing to PMT, stress would appear to be a strong mediating factor. Whether the pressure is at work or due to domestic or social circumstances, our reproductive cycles can be profoundly affected.

PMT may be so mild that you only barely notice certain changes in your body or yourself, or so severe that it interferes with work, with manual dexterity and threatens domestic happiness. The symptoms usually comprise an increase in breast size, breast tenderness, weight gain, abdominal distention, fluid retention, constipation or diarrhoea, increase in skin pigmentation, spots, depression, tearfulness, emotional outbursts, sugar craving leading to overeating, an increase in alcohol consumption, fatigue—and an increased need to sleep—but difficulty getting to sleep, aches and pains, and nausea.

How to Cope with PMT: Until the cause has been elucidated, treatment will be elusive, but there is much you can do to help yourself.

- **Start a menstrual calendar:** This will help you to pinpoint on any one day where you are in your cycle and what's going on in your body. Day 1 should be the first day of a period, day 14 is when you ovulate during a 28-day cycle. (Ovulation is *always* 14 days *before* your period, so, if your cycle is longer than 28 days subtract 14 to find out when you're ovulating.) Using letters or abbreviations, note down how you feel and whether your normal routines are disrupted.

- **Sleep more:** Use your calendar to work out when your PMT symptoms start, and make a point of going to bed earlier during that time. Treat yourself to at least two early nights. Have a long hot bath, shut the world out and take to your bed with a good book or magazine. You'll sleep soundly and awake feeling refreshed and regenerated.

- **Food** *Hypoglycaemia* The hunger pangs and sugar craving of premenstrual days are the result of low blood sugar. Eating chocolate and sweet things makes matters much worse. Eat wholefoods which are filling (as you eat less) yet good sources of carbohydrate which will release sugar gradually over a period of time. If you feel nauseous eat little and often.

  Constipation Eat wholefoods, rich in dietary fibre to prevent and help with constipation—which if not the cause of your bloated tummy, certainly won't make it feel better. Also drink sufficient fluid.

  Fluid retention Avoid salt (which attracts water) and eat naturally diuretic foods such as rhubarb, prunes, cucumber, celery. Also eat potassium-rich foods such as bananas, dried fruit, oranges and tomatoes.

  Vitamins and minerals There is research to show that women who suffer badly with PMT may be deficient in some or all of the following: vitamin B_6 (pyridoxine), vitamin E, calcium, magnesium and zinc. See p. 102 for the richest food sources.

- **Exercise:** Exercise can do much to prevent premenstrual tension. The mechanism for this is not clear but probably related to effective stress release and therefore preventing the build-up of certain hormones. Once you are in the premenstrual phase, it will be too late to reverse things totally, but you will find a relaxing jog or a long walk very calming. Resolve to start up our Basic Exercise Plan once your period has started (perhaps the second day) and note down your progress and how you feel on your menstrual calendar—you'll be surprised!

MAJOR BODY CHANGES

Contraception and Sport

There is no evidence that any form of contraception has a direct effect on sporting activity, but when choosing or changing your contraceptive method, you should take into account not only its effectiveness but also any health risks and known side effects involved. The Pill, chosen by many sportswomen for its hormone regulation and 100% reliability, carries considerable health risks for some women. Rhythm methods are medically safe, but have a high failure rate. Get comprehensive advice from your doctor before making your decision.

HORMONAL	INTRA-UTERINE DEVICE ('coil')	BARRIER	NATURAL/RHYTHM
Combined Pill Totally abolishes natural menstrual cycle. Regular cycle allows you to concentrate on your sport: no distraction because of pregnancy fears or painful or heavy periods. Doesn't necessarily prevent PMT and can make it worse. The fitter you are, the more easily tolerated are the side effects. Can mask subfertility problems — therefore, long-term use in amenorrhoeic women not recommended. **Progesterone-only Pill (POP or 'Mini-Pill')** Main action on cervical mucus rendering it hostile to sperm. Periods real, but may be very irregular at first. Breakthrough bleeds common. PMT very often relieved. Suitable for use while breast-feeding. **Injectables — eg, Depo-Provera, Noragest** Deep intramuscular injection of synthetic progesterone inhibits ovulation for 3 months. Not suitable while breast-feeding.	Foreign object in uterus sets up tissue reaction so implantation actively discouraged. Does not prevent fertilisation. IUDs come in many different shapes and sizes, and some are impregnated with copper. Newer and smaller designs now make this method available to women who have not had children. Abdominal cramps and pain common, particularly for first few cycles as uterus gets used to presence of coil. Discomfort can be exacerbated by exercise. Periods usually heavier, longer and more painful.	**Diaphragm ('Dutch cap') Cervical Cap (vimule)** Rubber dome-shaped device covers cervix to prevent entry by sperm. Should in no way hinder any sport or exercise. Any discomfort implies faulty insertion or wrong fitting. Because of proximity to bladder, can cause frequency of urine and exacerbate cystitis. **Sheath** Very fine rubber 'stocking' fitted onto erect penis long before penetration. Impregnated with spermicide. Strictly speaking, effect on sport none, since used by male. May react 'allergically' to spermicide — eg, rash on thighs or persistent burning sensation internally. **Sponge** Large 'marshmallow' sponge impregnated with spermicide. No effect on sport. **Spermicide** Despite name, main action is immobilising rather than killing sperm. Inevitable dribbling so wear panty-liners. Allergic reaction and/or fungal infection common.	**Calendar** From date of previous period can calculate date of next and, by subtracting 14 days, probable date of ovulation. **Temperature** Body temperature taken every morning. Sudden drop indicates ovulation and intercourse should be avoided. **Muco-thermal** Colour and consistency of cervical mucus indicates pre- and post-ovulation phases of cycle. Women who are more physically active may be more in tune with their bodies and therefore make much shrewder judgements as to when ovulation is about to take place. However, some active women may find that exercise has disrupted their menstrual cycle, and so they cannot use this method effectively.

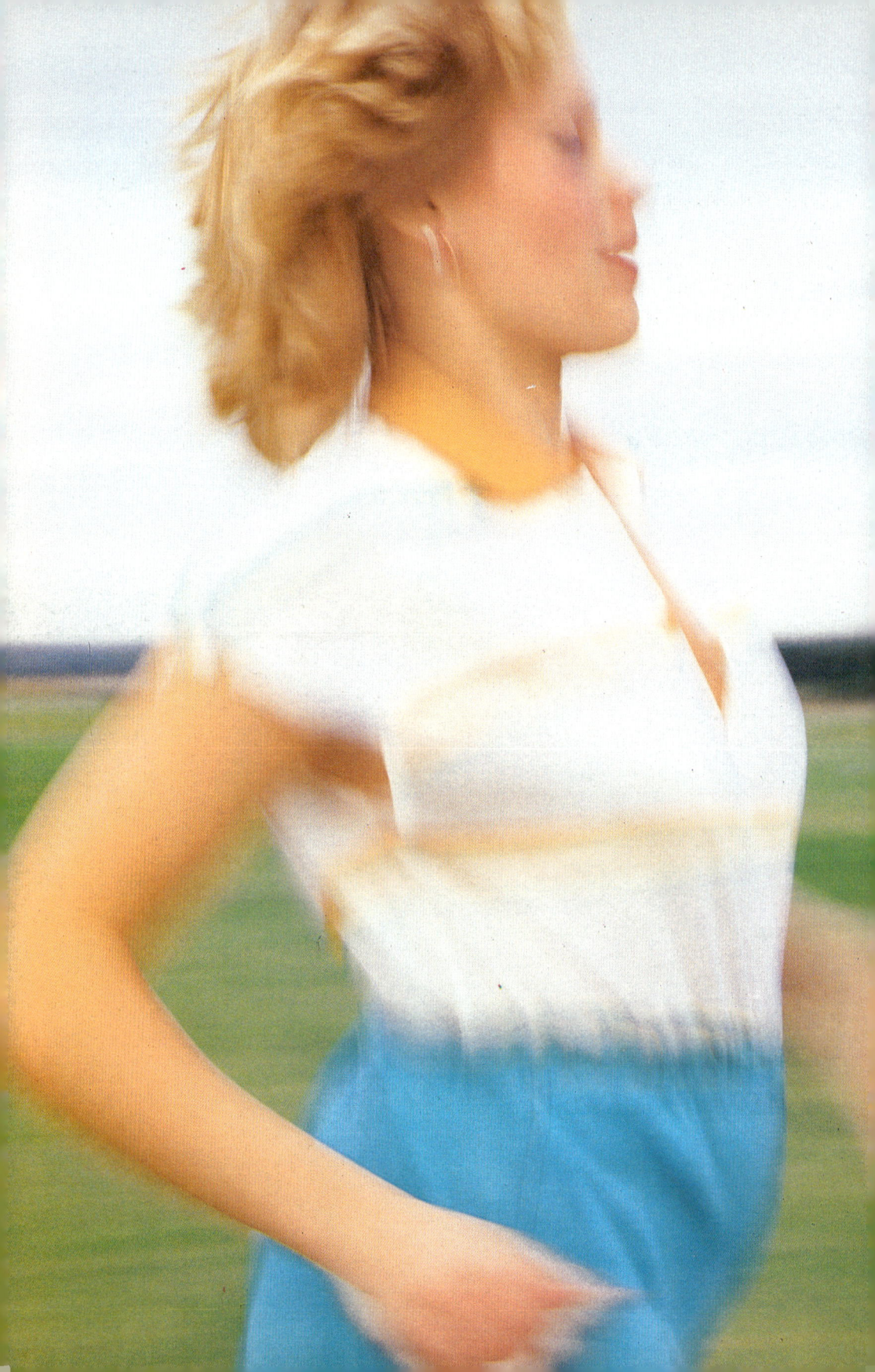

MAJOR BODY CHANGES

Pregnancy

Traditionally, this was a time to put your feet up and take it easy. Nowadays we know the benefits of staying active during pregnancy. A fit mother copes with the ups and downs of pregnancy better, has an easier labour, fewer complications, and far less chance of Caesarian delivery. Nevertheless, it is important to realise that pregnancy will make unusual demands on your body and from very early on you will probably want to consider some special needs including more sleep, a good, wholesome diet, psychological support, rest and relaxation, exercise for perking-up and stamina and exercises for muscle-toning.

MAJOR BODY CHANGES

Getting Fit for Pregnancy

Like any other major event, the nine months of pregnancy, the birth and subsequent recovery are all much easier if you are healthy and fit and your muscles are in trim and ready to work hard. It's never too late to get fit and if you plan to have a baby, then plan to get fit at the same time (see pp. 84–5). Once you are pregnant, it is often too late to reach a high level of fitness, although there is much you can do to get fitter (see p. 84).

Your muscles will need to be both strong and flexible—especially the abdominal muscles which will have to carry the baby. If these muscles are weak, then the muscles of the lower back will have to take on extra duties—and the result, very often, is the 'classic' lower back pain of pregnancy. (See exercises opposite and tips on posture on p. 76.)

Preparing to Have a Baby

Babies do not always begin when you want them to. Getting pregnant is not always just a matter of stopping whatever form of contraception you have been using and starting straight away. Some women do conceive immediately, others—for a variety of reasons—do not and get anxious as the months go by, reducing their chances still more. A good diet, no tobacco, only very moderate alcohol, and a sensible fitness programme (preferably for your partner as well) will help ensure that your body is in good health and is more relaxed. This will increase your chances of conception as well as getting the eventual pregnancy off to a good start. When there is a delay in getting pregnant, many doctors often recommend a holiday or similar break as anxiety can inhibit conception. Not many of us can think in those terms, but an hour's sport or exercise, say three times a week, that gets both of you 'away from it all' may prove surprisingly effective.

Healthy Habits: In the past, no one ever gave much thought to preparing to have a child—certainly not in the manner just outlined or in terms of fitness. This approach to pregnancy is very much a product of the 1980s—as ante-natal care was of the 1920s. So, although your mother may have taken no special exercise in pregnancy, smoked, and eaten for two, it doesn't entitle you to do the same.

Habits of poor eating, drinking alcohol and smoking are difficult to change, but if you and your partner resolve to get the pregnancy and your child off to the best possible start, then hopefully you can encourage one another to cut back on one of these vices—or stop them altogether. Very often, one healthy habit leads to another and if you resolve to improve your fitness you will naturally begin to care about what you eat (see Nutrition and Diet p. 90) and to avoid anything which risks harming you, your chances of conceiving, or the foetus.

Check List

Although some of the following conditions cannot be ascertained until the pregnancy is fairly advanced, you should be cautious about strenuous exercise and consult your doctor if you have:

- Heart disease
- Diabetes or 'gestational diabetes'
- An incompetent cervix
- *Any* abdominal pain or cramps
- A history of two, three or more miscarriages
- *Any* vaginal bleeding—at *any* stage in pregnancy
- Marked ankle swelling
- High blood pressure
- Twin or triplet (or more!) pregnancy
- Ruptured membranes.

MAJOR BODY CHANGES

Stretching in Pregnancy

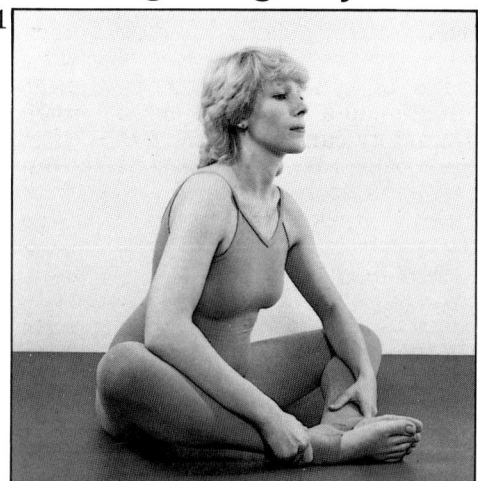

1 Inner Thigh Stretch
Sitting on floor with soles of feet together, clasp ankles, and with elbows resting on knees, press legs slowly down to floor. Hold for count of 10. Keep back straight.

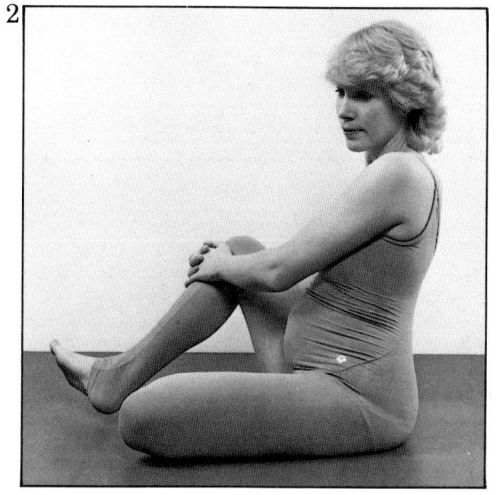

2 Ankle Strengthener
Resting on coccyx (sitting bone) with left leg bent under you, clasp right knee and rotate foot to right making exaggerated circle. Do 5 times, then repeat rotation to left 5 times. Repeat with other foot and rotate in both directions 5 times.

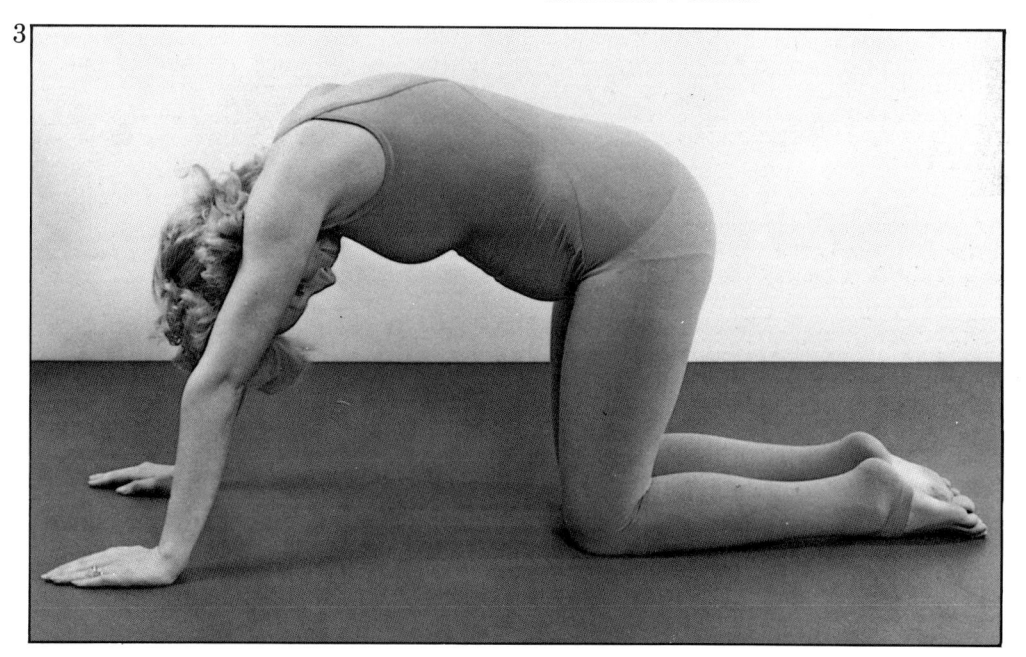

3 Aching Back Stretch
Kneel on all-fours with your weight evenly distributed. Make sure your back is straight and doesn't sag. Hold. Gradually raise your back, dropping head and shoulders, and breathe out. Tighten pelvic floor and bottom muscles. Hold, then relax gently. Never allow back to sag. Repeat 5 times.

MAJOR BODY CHANGES

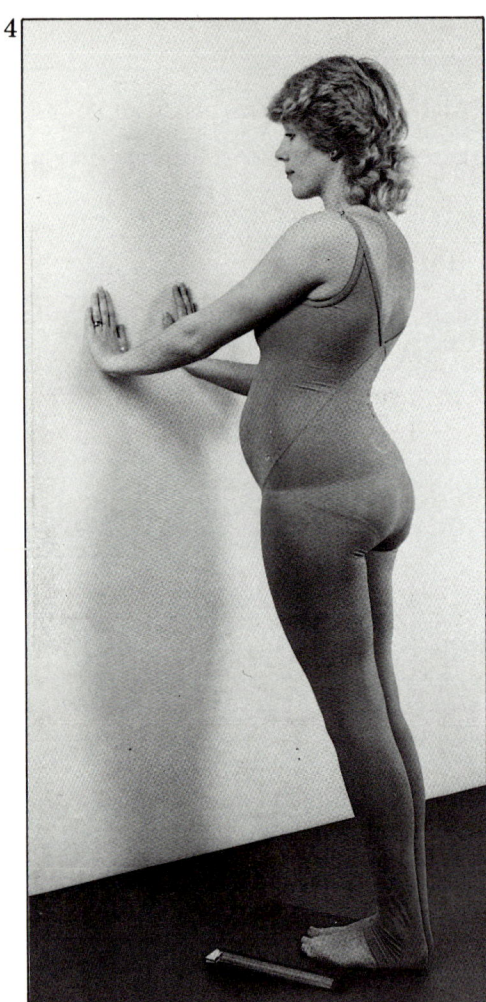

4 Calf and Tendon Stretch
Calf: Stand on a large book with hand resting against wall. Gently raise yourself on balls of feet and hold for a count of 5. Lower slowly. Repeat 4 times.

Tendon: Stand on large book with heels hanging over edge. Lower heels to floor and feel stretch. Hold for count of 10 and repeat.

5 Waist Stretch
Standing with feet hip-width apart and left foot turned slightly outwards, raise and extend arms outwards at shoulder level. Slowly bend over and reach for left foot, holding right arm straight above. Gently straighten yourself and repeat on other side.

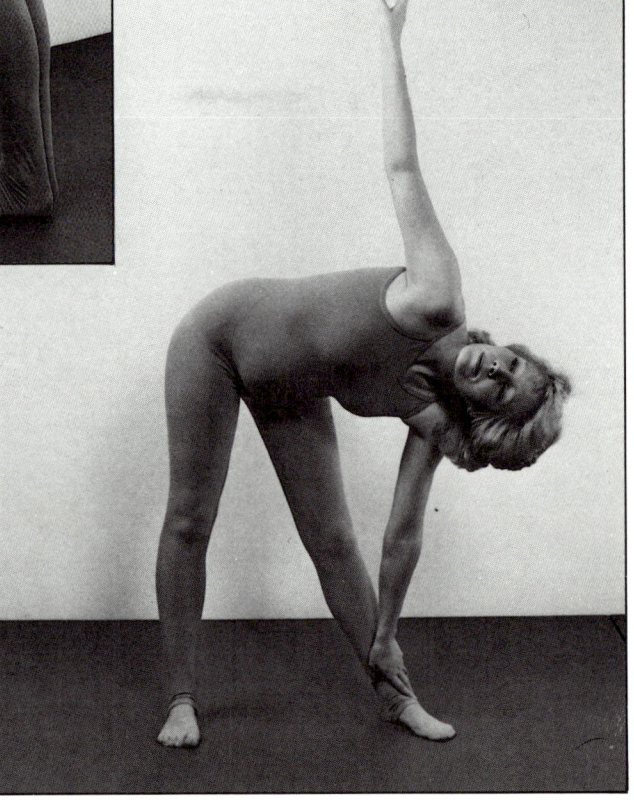

MAJOR BODY CHANGES

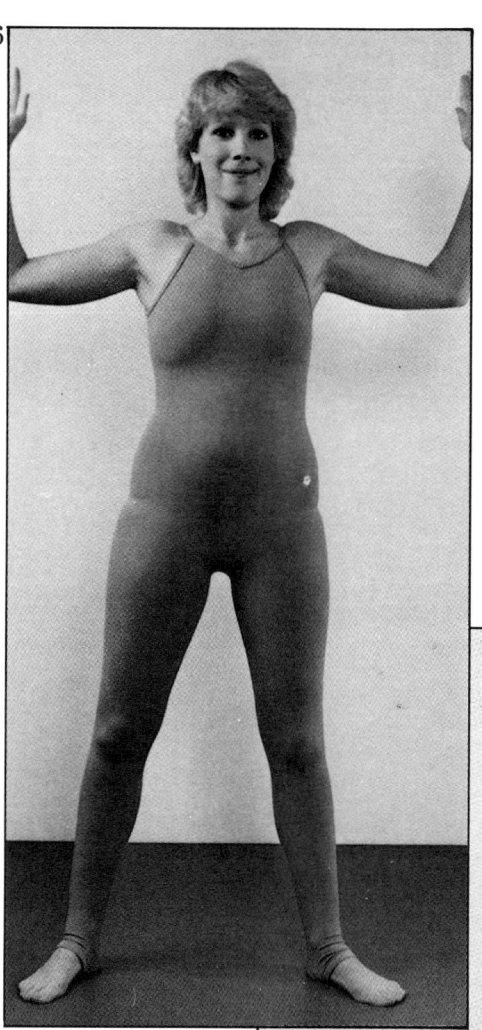

6 Breast and Pectoral Muscle Toner
Standing with feet hip-width apart, raise arms to shoulder level, bent at elbows, and breathe in. Breathing out, bring arms to centre so that forearms touch. Breathe in and open arms out again. Repeat 5 times.

7 Hip Swing
Standing with left foot on large book and left hand against wall, gently swing right leg forwards (lifting no higher than 45° angle). Do this 10 times, swing leg to side 10 times, swing leg back 10 times.

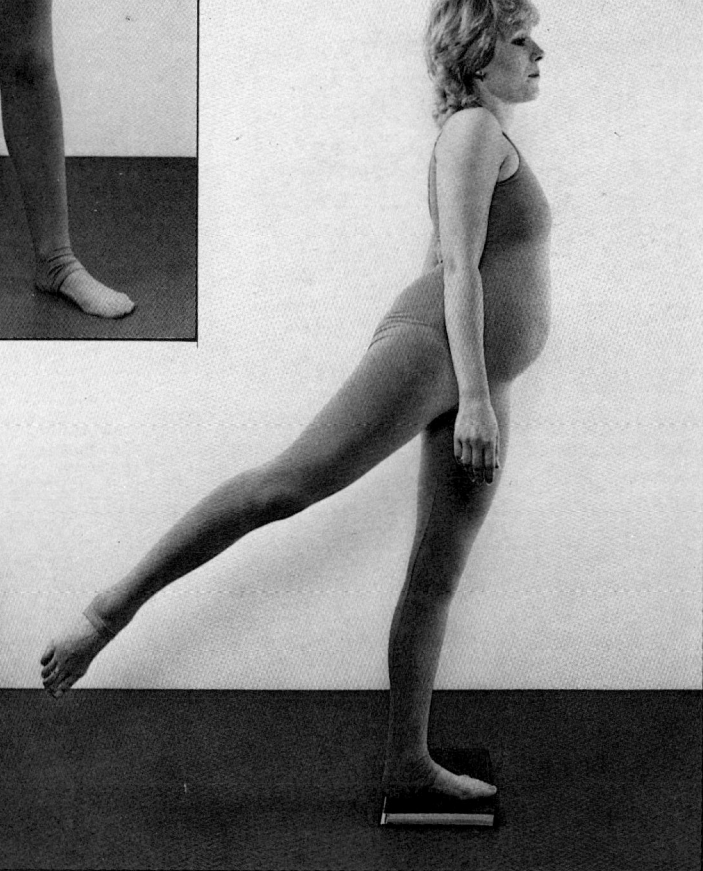

MAJOR BODY CHANGES

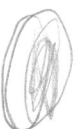

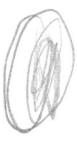

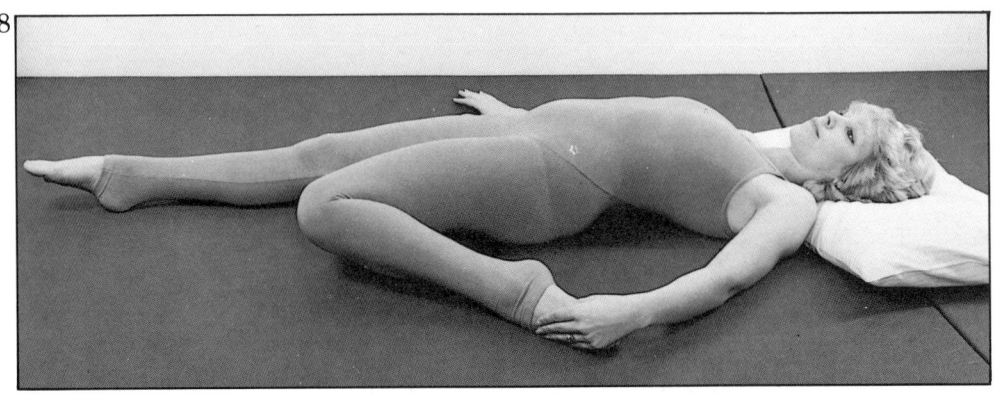

8 Thigh Stretch
Lying on your back, gently bend left leg out to side and hold toes with left hand. Hold stretch for count of 15. Don't force, as this risks knee stress. Repeat with left leg.

9 Bottom Firmer
Keeping feet flat and shoulders on floor, raise hips off the floor gradually, squeezing your pelvic floor and bottom muscles. Hold for count of 5, then slowly release muscles as you lower hips.

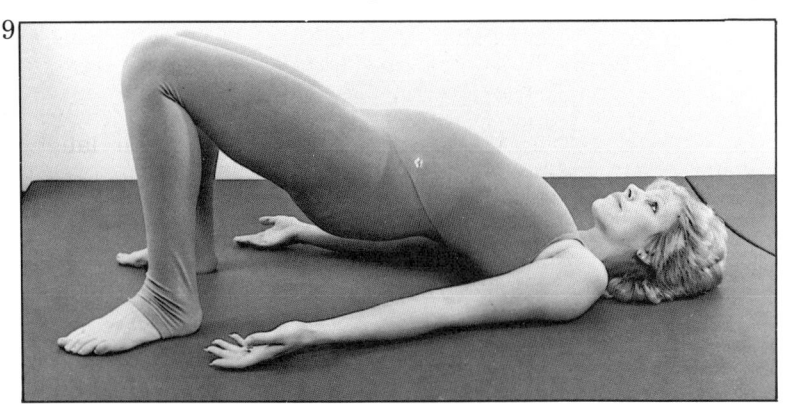

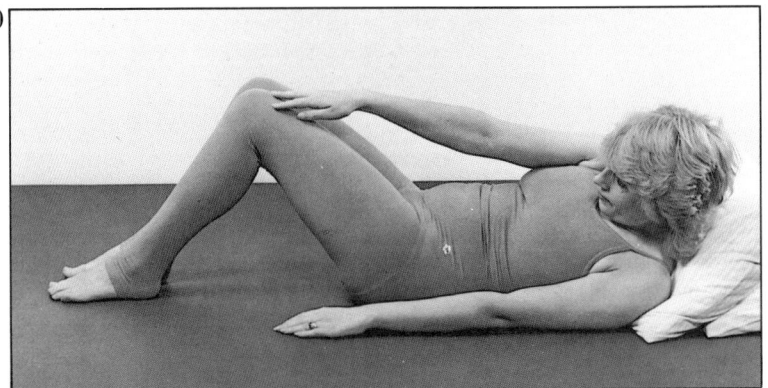

10 Tummy Muscle Toner
Lie on your back with knees bent and feet flat on the floor. Lift your head and shoulder slightly and with left hand reach out and touch right knee. Lower yourself to the floor and repeat on the other side. Do 5 times on each side at first, gradually building up to 10 times daily. Do not attempt this exercise with legs straight.

Exercise during Pregnancy

Also see Code for exercise in pregnancy in Sport and Exercise Guide.

When to Begin

Basically, the first three months (trimester) are when you are—and feel—most vulnerable; the second three months when you feel best; and the third three months when you feel—and most likely are—most awkward. Given this, you won't want to start doing anything too energetic in the first months unless your body is well and truly used to regular exercise, and you simply won't be able to in the last couple of months before the baby is born. So, unless you are something of a sportswoman you should look to the second trimester as the time to undertake a serious disciplined approach to toning up your body for labour and delivery while gradually warming up in the 1st trimester with walks, plus stretching exercises. Giving birth is an endurance event, and the fitter you are physically and psychologically (strong arms and thighs, a firmed up pelvic floor, some heart-lung stamina and calm of mind) the better you will feel, the better you'll be able to actively take part in the birth process and the better recovery you'll make afterwards.

What to Wear: If you already have some sport or exercise gear and a sports bra, this will probably do you until *about* 12 weeks. If you don't, you might like to consider borrowing your partner's tracksuit bottoms, T-shirts etc before deciding if you want to buy anything new. Sports bras, however, are strongly recommended and should be one or two sizes up from your normal bra size. For later in pregnancy (and also breastfeeding), you might like to consider a comfortable and supporting pregnancy/nursing bra with ties at the back which can be loosened as your rib cage expands in the last trimester, and tightened again after delivery. As for clothes, buy whatever you feel—and will continue to feel—very comfortable in, one or two sizes up. Shoes—see p. 31.

The First Trimester

You may feel over the moon, or under the weather; chances are, you feel a bit of both depending on many things and not least, the time of day. Not everyone is plagued by morning sickness, but you will probably feel nauseous at some point (some women are sick at night) and 'go off' certain things—notably, alcohol, cigarettes, tea and coffee. This and many other 'quirks' of pregnancy are normal and hormonal in origin and a sign of the enormous changes taking place in your body as the foetus settles in. Apart from these physical symptoms, there may be mental ones too: you feel extremely and perpetually tired and just want to sleep (try to grab forty-winks during the day or catch up with long lie-ins at weekends), perhaps you feel slightly disorientated, drop things, feel light-headed and that your sense of balance is slightly upset; or you burst into laughter or tears for no explicable reason and you question and wonder 'Am I ready for this?' All these feelings are normal—not least, those of ambivalence. But whatever you feel—and whether you spend most of the day stuck at home or stuck in an office—it is important to set aside a certain amount of time each day to actively concentrate on your needs. Do some gently stretching exercises (p. 69) when you get up (or once the nausea has subsided), and do go for a walk (15–30 mins) every day—preferably without youngsters or shopping. Also try some gentle, relaxing swimming. All this is not only good for your circulation and muscle-toning, but can be a great psychological boost too. Even if you don't feel up to much, do take time out to 'get away from it all' in your mind, and gently exercise your body at the same time. It'll work wonders in helping you fight off the nausea, any bizarre cravings and any dark thoughts.

The Second Trimester

Don't panic around 24 weeks if your pulse seems to be thundering along at a quicker pace. It is. However, the cardiac output is at its highest between 25 and 28 weeks which may be a time to make especially sure that you don't overdo it.

Remember the aim of exercise at this time is to keep the body mobile and active, to maintain the positive health benefits and to be in good shape again after birth. Go for comfortable and enjoyable exercise—not a hard workout.

After five months, it begins to become harder to move around. Not only is your tummy increasing, but also your blood takes longer to pump back from extremities (hands, feet) past the uterus. So, if your body says it's hard work doing regular sports, switch to ones where the load is spread more comfortably—cycling (but not in heavy traffic!) and swimming are both *supported* forms of movement.

Of course there will be times when you need more rest. Try to build this into a timetable and try out the relaxation techniques outlined in the chapter on p.111. There are also times when exercise is not advisable—see p. 68.

The Benefits of Good Posture

The benefits of good posture are manifold: You feel better; you are better able to expand your rib cage and to breathe freely; your shoulders are relaxed, avoiding muscle tension; your spine lengthens so the baby has more room; your abdominal muscles are actively used to support the baby and so quickly regain their tone after delivery; and because your pelvis is centred, you can make full use of your abdominal and buttock muscles and so prevent back strain.

Bad posture is easily encouraged by the weight of the baby, tilting of the pelvis, and poor muscle tone. If your stomach and buttock muscles are not used to support the baby (like a corset), there is a tendency to overarch the back to compensate for the extra weight at the front; your stomach, bottom and thighs can't work properly and so lose their tone.

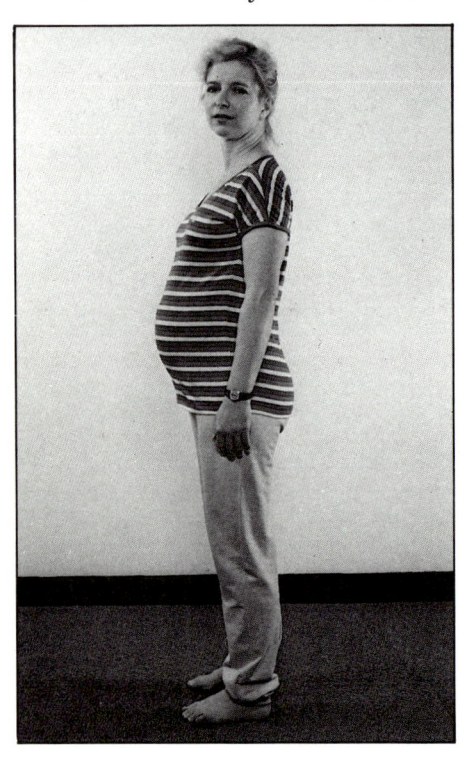

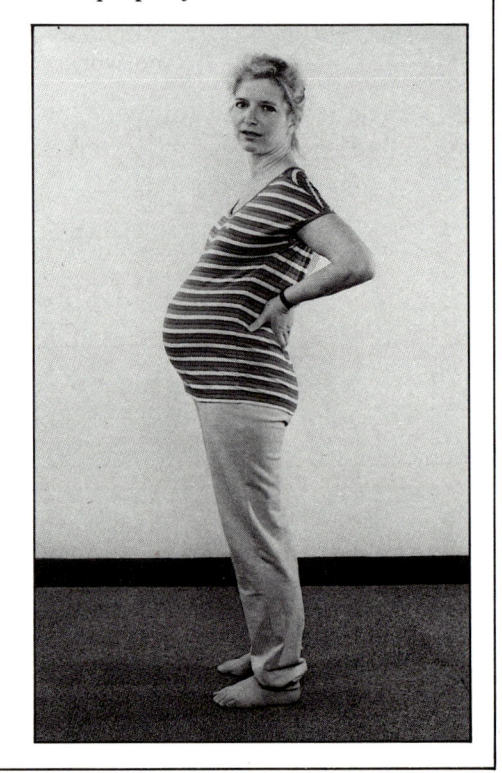

MAJOR BODY CHANGES

The Third Trimester

By now, even housework is getting awkward because it does involve a lot of standing and bending down. However, try squatting instead of bending; this will help open up and tone the pelvic floor area and is more comfortable and better for your back than stooping. Specific exercises to tone muscles (see p. 80) are particularly valuable now, so don't give up!

More and more active women are reporting that they have continued enjoying sport until the last few weeks of pregnancy. Swimming especially, can be enjoyed right up to delivery! However, certain sports—eg, alpine skiing, riding, judo etc are not recommended now as you are more prone to falls and injury. One cross-country ski champion gave up skiing after 8 months: 'because I couldn't get up again after I fell over—the bump got in the way!'

From about 32 weeks, you will be feeling increasingly tired so follow your instincts and *do* rest more.

When to Stop

There are regular joggers who boast of continuing until their seventh or eighth month, but, interestingly, the world's fastest marathon runner, Ingrid Kristiansen of Norway, switched to cycling and swimming after eight months 'to take the weight off my feet'. In fact the 27-year-old was four months pregnant when she ran in the world cross-country championships in 1983—without realising it. She was a classic example of a top-class athlete with amenorrhoea (see p. 63) but still fertile. After a 3½-hour labour she gave birth to a healthy son and was running (very gently) ten days later.

However, not everyone—serious sportswoman or not—is able to continue with their sport or exercise programme throughout pregnancy. For whatever reason—immediate weight gain, fatigue, shortness of breath—some women find that they cannot keep going; they have to cut right back on their mileage or switch to less demanding forms of exercise very early on in pregnancy. There is no way of telling beforehand how your body will react to pregnancy—everyone is

Injuries

Sport and exercise injuries are a nuisance at the best of times but if sustained during pregnancy, they're really no joke. Consider the following and you'll understand why:

- No pain-killing or anti-inflammatory drugs should be taken for strains or sprains without full consultation with your doctor. This is particularly important in the first and second trimesters.

- No X-rays can be performed to diagnose broken bones etc until about 36 weeks (4 weeks before the baby is due) when the risk to the baby is minimal.

- As your pregnancy advances, your enlarging tummy alters your centre of gravity and therefore sense of balance, and in the third trimester, the hormone relaxin loosens your muscles and ligaments and you are therefore at an increased risk of falls and injury.

- For serious injuries, the need to use anaesthetics and strong analgesia to set bones etc will be weighed against the possible risks to your baby.

So, do be careful. For more information on the treatment and prevention of injuries, see p. 50.

different and every pregnancy you go through is different.

Don't give up without trying at least, but *do listen to your body*. When it says 'stop!' then stop, and take up swimming and walking instead. There are also certain conditions and signs which demand that you pass up on strenuous physical activity (see table).

Common Anxieties

There are many fears and anxieties concerning exercise in pregnancy—many of them unfounded and based on hearsay or old wives' tales. The baby is well protected from the outside world by

MAJOR BODY CHANGES

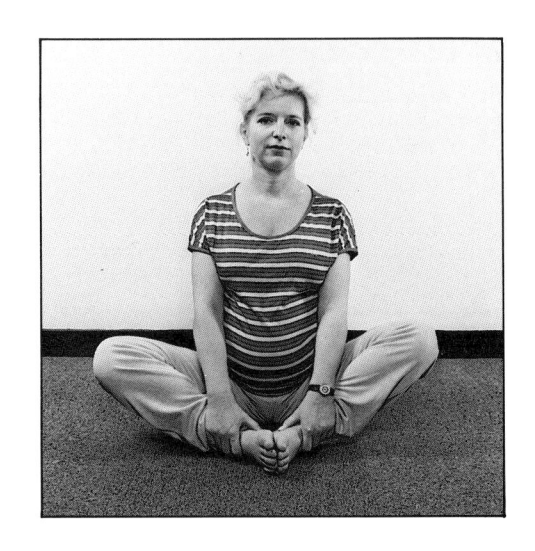

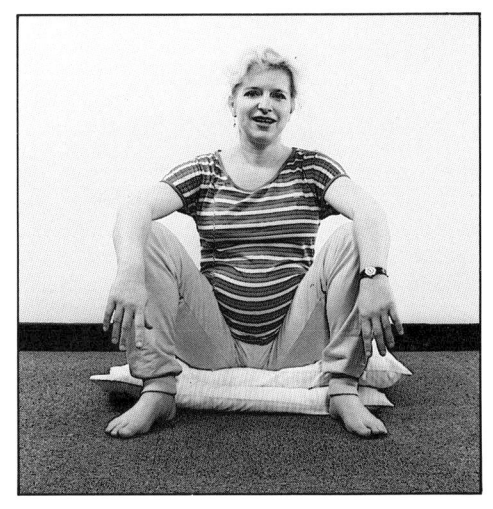

Sitting Comfortably

Below are comfortable positions for sitting which open up the chest and pelvic area and encourage a straight back. Unlike sitting in a chair, there is less tendency towards bad posture such as slouching or crossing legs which can cause cramp and exacerbate varicose veins. At first try sitting up against a wall so that you learn to feel when your back is straight. You should be able to feel the length of your spine pressing into the wall. Then try sitting unsupported with feet pressed together or legs wide apart as shown.

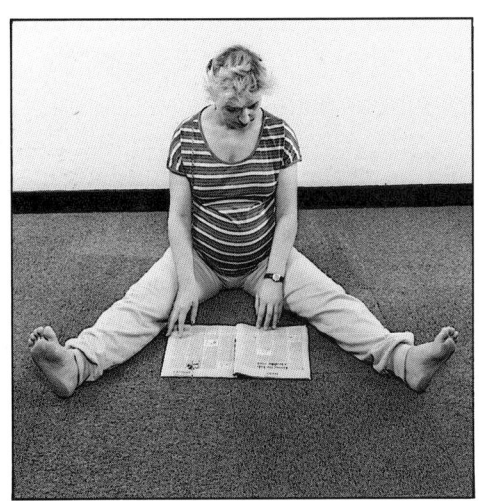

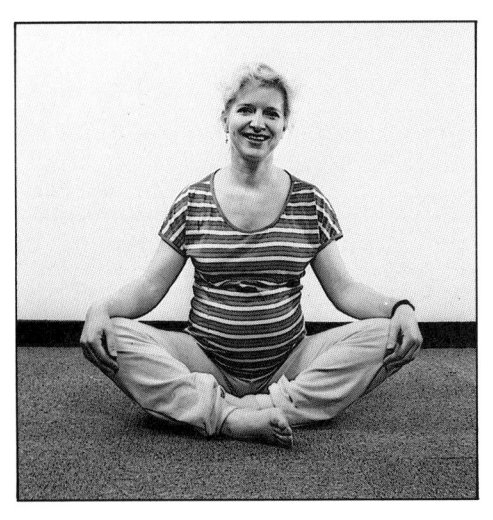

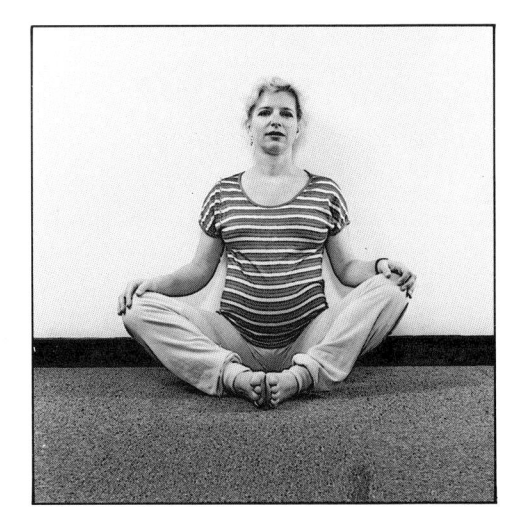

MAJOR BODY CHANGES

Moving Comfortably

1 Squatting This is preferable to bending and stooping, and comfortable for doing housework or when playing with children or talking on the phone. It makes use of thigh muscles and opens up the pelvic area.
2 Lifting Keeping feet firmly flat on floor, bend knees and keep back straight; placing one foot in front of the other will give you more stability.
3 Lying Down A relaxing position for resting, opening up the pelvic area; place small cushion in lower back.
4 Getting Up and Lying Down Turn onto your side, rest on hip and pause while your circulation adjusts to change in posture.

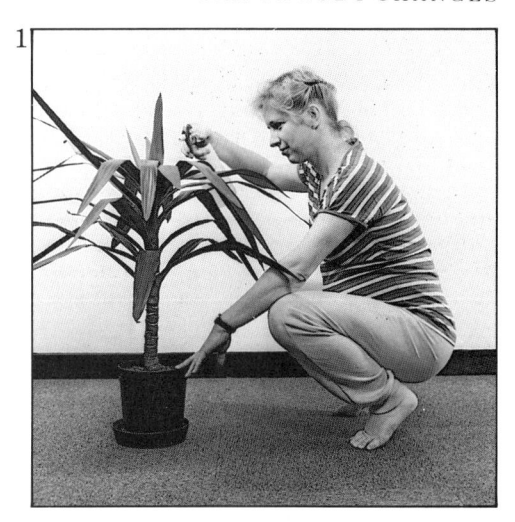

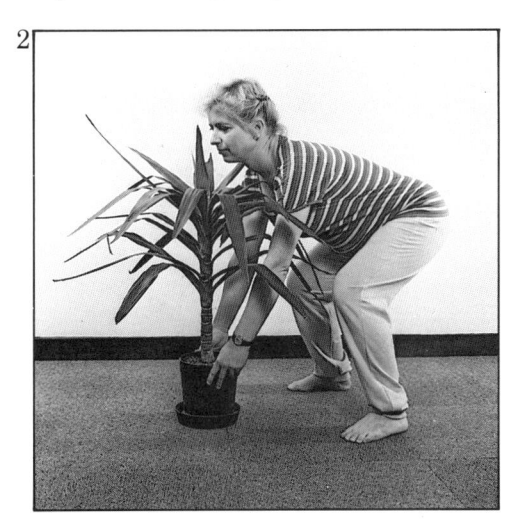

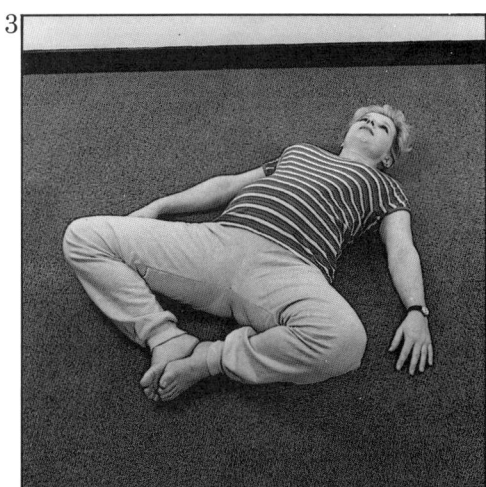

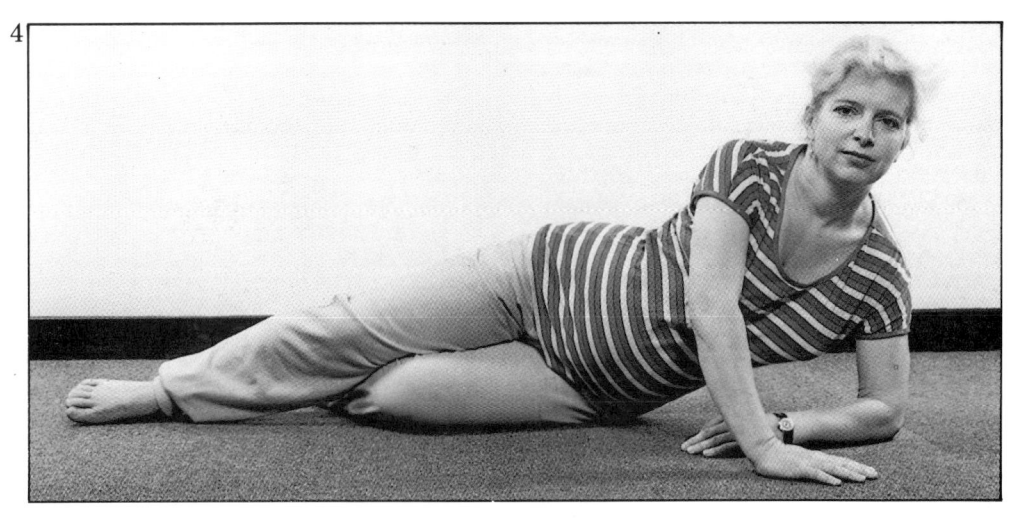

a large bag which is full of sterile fluid (amniotic fluid), and this in turn lies within the uterus. It is the amniotic fluid in which the baby floats—and is lulled to sleep when you are active—that cushions it from knocks and jostles. It would take a severe and direct blow to the abdomen to do any harm.

Miscarriage: There has always been a fear that exercise of any kind (let alone sport) would cause a spontaneous abortion. The first three months have always been regarded (and rightly so) as the most risky time, as the foetus settles in. However, all research comes up with the same answer: the rate of miscarriage in active and inactive women is exactly the same—ie, of confirmed pregnancies, 25% miscarry, and of early undiagnosed pregnancies, 75% miscarry—and that a miscarriage is Nature's way of ensuring that only healthy foetuses are allowed to develop to term. More significant perhaps, is the argument that women who take an active, regular part in sport are *less likely* to miscarry than their sedentary sisters since they will probably be non-smokers, moderate drinkers and sensible eaters—all factors which affect not only the chances of conception but also the viability of the foetus.

If a miscarriage does, sadly, take place, you might find that exercise is a good way of venting your grief and anger. It will also give you the resolve to look after yourself and give you the courage to try again when you feel ready.

Swimming and Infection: Another classic fear is that swimming will cause infection to reach the baby. Theoretically, this is not possible as the cervix (neck of the womb) is sealed with a plug of mucus. However, towards the very end of pregnancy—especially in women who have borne children before—the cervix will begin to dilate, although the mucus plug is still in place. Strictly speaking, these women are slightly at risk of allowing possible infection to ascend through the cervix even though the bag of waters is still intact. Women who should *not swim* (or even have a bath) are those who have any vaginal bleeding, have had a 'show'

or whose waters have broken. Apart from these instances, swimming in a pool (both cleaner and safer than swimming in the sea) is quite safe in pregnancy and a very good form of exercise and relaxation.

Depriving the Baby of Oxygen: One of the physiological effects of pregnancy is breathlessness. This is partly due to the hormone progesterone acting on the brain's respiratory receptors and partly, if not mostly, due to the baby pressing on and lifting the diaphragm —which retards full expansion of the lungs. (Another reason for breathlessness might be anaemia). However, it has been argued that in addition to this, the 'puffing and panting' that comes with exercise serves only to make the mother even more breathless and so deprive the baby of oxygen. The fact is, some women become more breathless than others and may therefore find certain forms of exercise trying—in which case they should switch to a more gentle form of workout—while the baby takes all the oxygen it needs from the mother. It is only in cases where the mother's breathing is already laboured because of serious illness (heart disease, respiratory disease, heavy smoking, severe anaemia) that the baby is at risk. What is more, since exercise stimulates the mother's circulation, the baby actually receives more—and better-oxygenated—blood than it might otherwise.

Weight Gain

Weight gain is inevitable in pregnancy. The total amount of weight gained will vary from one woman to another and from one pregnancy to another, but is generally in the region of 20–30 lbs (9–13½ kg). There is no hard and fast rule about how much weight you should gain and at what rate, although a rate of about ½ lb (250 g) per week for the first four months doubling for the next three, and then settling down is probably about right. Insufficient weight gain is associated with just as many—and often more serious—problems as excess weight gain. But the weight you gain is not all fat, it comprises the weight of the baby, the amniotic fluid, the placenta,

Stride Jumps (after the birth)

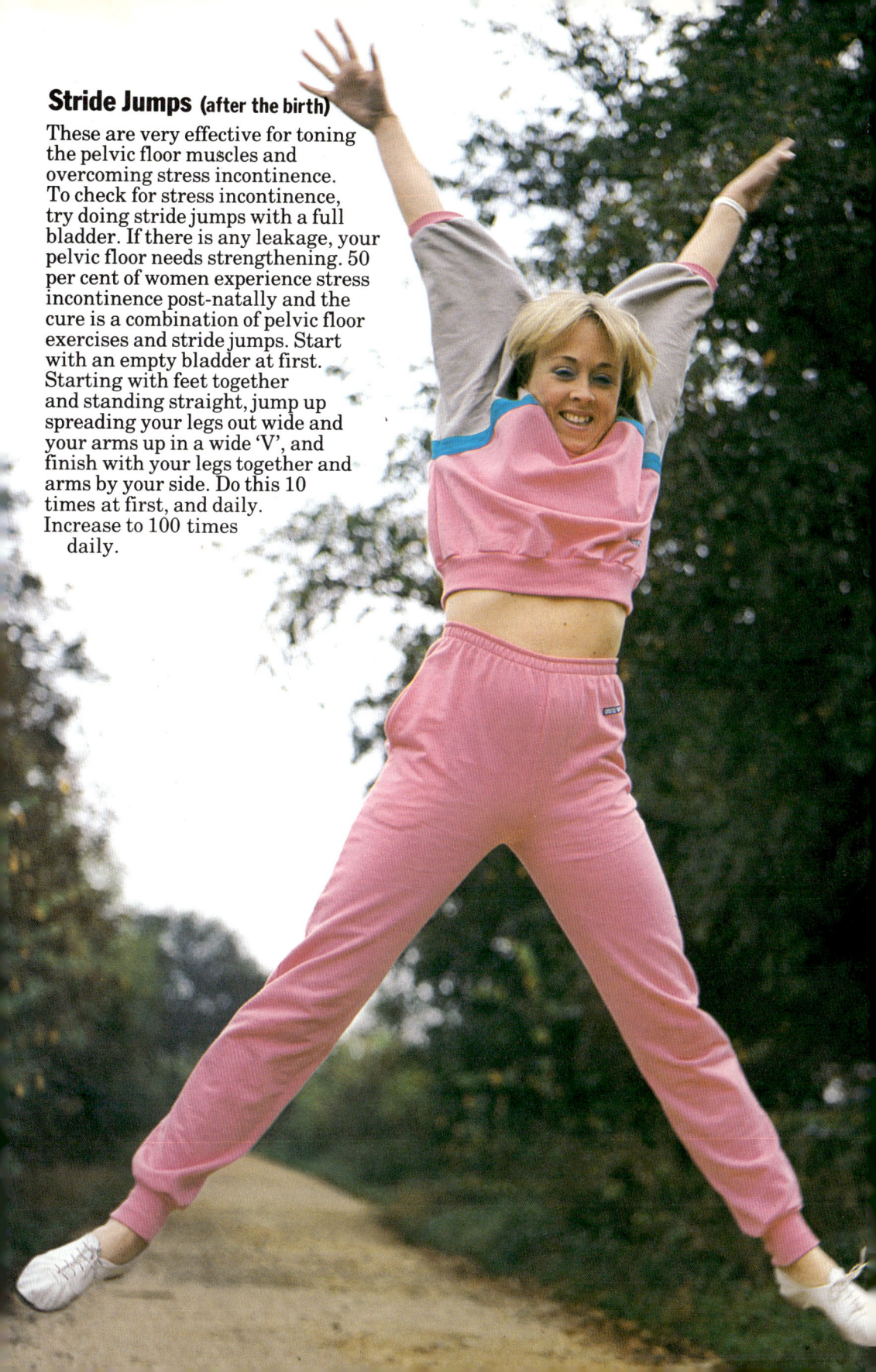

These are very effective for toning the pelvic floor muscles and overcoming stress incontinence. To check for stress incontinence, try doing stride jumps with a full bladder. If there is any leakage, your pelvic floor needs strengthening. 50 per cent of women experience stress incontinence post-natally and the cure is a combination of pelvic floor exercises and stride jumps. Start with an empty bladder at first. Starting with feet together and standing straight, jump up spreading your legs out wide and your arms up in a wide 'V', and finish with your legs together and arms by your side. Do this 10 times at first, and daily. Increase to 100 times daily.

MAJOR BODY CHANGES

your enlarged uterus, the tissue, fluid and colostrum in your breasts, the increase in blood volume, and the extra fat laid down for breast feeding.

While many experts say that you should notice no alteration in weight during the first trimester, for many women this simply is not the case and probably reflects the fact that you are not usually seen or weighed by a doctor or clinic before twelve weeks. Some women note a change in their shape and weight gain within weeks of conception; others—because of nausea or vomiting—actually lose weight. This is not really desirable and the sooner their weight stabilises and begins to increase, the better. If you think you're gaining weight rather too quickly, take a hard look at what you're eating and turn to the chapter on nutrition and diet on p. 90 . Whatever you do, don't stop

Pelvic Floor Muscles

These muscles exist in both men and women, but are of more significance to a woman's health because they cradle the pelvic structures. Unlike the obvious muscles of the arms and legs, or even the easily locatable 'hidden' muscles of the stomach or back, these muscles are 'inside', wrapped like a figure of 8 around the anus, urinary opening and vagina. Also described as a hammock-like web of muscles supporting the inside of the pelvis, the muscles are used when going to the toilet, for sex, during pregnancy, for giving birth, as well as reacting to coughs and sneezes, laughing and lifting objects and orgasm. They are important throughout a woman's life, and should be kept in trim for optimum health.

Identifying the Muscles

The easiest way is to try to stop urinating when you are on the toilet. If you can stop in midstream, you are using your pelvic floor muscles. Another way of identifying them is to insert your finger into your vagina and then try to 'squeeze' it; better still, try 'squeezing' your partner's penis. If this is difficult, or he does not feel anything, then your muscles need toning.

Pelvic Floor Exercises

Try these while sitting squarely and comfortably on a firm chair, knees apart, and lean forward with your elbows on your knees, perhaps holding a book. Concentrate on contracting the correct muscles—not the stomach or thigh muscles. You may tire quite quickly at first but persist by doing a few contractions every hour, spread over a day.

1. Contract (that is, 'squeeze') the muscle for three seconds, then relax for five seconds. Breathe in as you contract; out as you relax. Do 25 times a day at first; building up to 50 times a day.

2. Contract and relax your pelvic floor muscles quickly, as quickly as you can but breathe *steadily*, not in time to the contractions. Do 25 times a day at first, then build up to 50 times a day. Do these anywhere: while on the phone or waiting for a cab or bus or watching TV.

3. Eventually your muscles will be well-toned enough to try the 'pelvic lift'. As well as contracting the muscle, try *pulling it upwards* as you breathe in. The effect is rather like that of an elevator or lift. At first, you will only be able to go up one or two floors, eventually, you will feel as if this internal elevator is shooting up several floors. The difficulty is in isolating these internal muscles, but practice makes it possible. Do 10 times a day, build up to 25 times a day.

4. Just as you get the lift to go up, you can practise 'going down', trying to urinate in a hurry or imagine trying to push something out of your vagina. Do 10 times a day; build up to 25 times a day.

eating or go on any crazy—especially low-calorie—diets. Pregnancy is not a time to start losing weight—the risks to your baby's health are not worth it.

If you eat sensibly, avoiding giving in too often to sweet food cravings, and avoid altogether high-calorie but nutritionally empty snacks, you shouldn't worry too much. A relatively high fibre diet is best because the dense food satisfies your hunger sooner and more effectively, and the fibre itself helps with constipation which is a physiological side effect of pregnancy. That being said, you may find salads and fruit and vegetables impossible to face in the first months. In this case, be imaginative: add bran to your soups and stews, bake wholemeal cookies—buy a wholesome cookery book!

Incidentally, the rationale behind exercise in pregnancy is *not* to lose weight or even keep weight gain in check. It is to tone up muscles, improve your heart/lung stamina, and to refresh and relax you. The fact it may also curb your appetite and make you more discerning about what you eat is simply an added bonus!

How do you Feel?

Your feelings about your body are an important part of your sexual identity and the way in which you present yourself to the world. (And what stronger symbol of sexuality than pregnancy?) Some women feel very proud, sexy and body conscious during pregnancy, but this isn't true of everyone—particularly in the last few weeks when you inevitably feel large and heavy. However, since we live in a society that knocks the natural female form and is perpetually trying to re-shape us according to some androgenous model, it is perhaps not surprising that some women don't greet their changing bodies positively. Dance and exercise is a superb way of putting you in touch with your body, allowing the natural release and expression of body feeling. It is also a great pick-me-up and a psychological boost on days when you're feeling low. Clothes too are important. Be imaginative, buy 'normal' clothes that you like, but one or two sizes larger, rather than hiding yourself in a tent!

After the Birth

Feeling low or slightly depressed after the baby is born is very common and natural. Not only is there a sudden drop in hormones, but you are consciously or unconsciously mourning the loss of the being nurtured inside you for nine whole months. The baby you carried and the baby delivered into your arms are frequently very different: since one was partly fantasy the baby you hold in your arms may well be strangely disappointing.

Close body and eye contact *immediately* after birth rekindles the bond between mother and child that was so rudely interrupted at delivery. Rather like imprinting in animals, the strength of maternal affection stems greatly from the quality and quantity of contact in those first precious days.

It is interesting to note that post-natal depression is higher among women who delivered in hospital than at home, and in those mothers who were not able to leave hospital soon after the birth. For them, the noisy and fussy hospital with all the alien faces and customs would seem to threaten the mother-child bond and can seriously undermine a mother's trust in her own instincts.

When you consider the effort involved and the energy expended during labour, it is not surprising that many women feel totally exhausted after delivery. The demands of a new baby in the first few days and weeks will also make you feel very tired. However, it is important to get back into—or start—some form of exercise as soon as possible, not only to tone up your stomach and pelvic floor muscles (opposite) but also give yourself more energy, strength and psychological support. Many women who exercised during pregnancy find that they are super-fit after delivery and can run twice as fast or perform twice as well as before. Exercise during pregnancy could therefore be regarded as a form of training as you are carrying extra weight about with you and your lungs and heart have to work extra hard. Once the baby is born, you will find it difficult to find the time to workout, but you must *make* the time.

MAJOR BODY CHANGES
Post-Natal Exercises

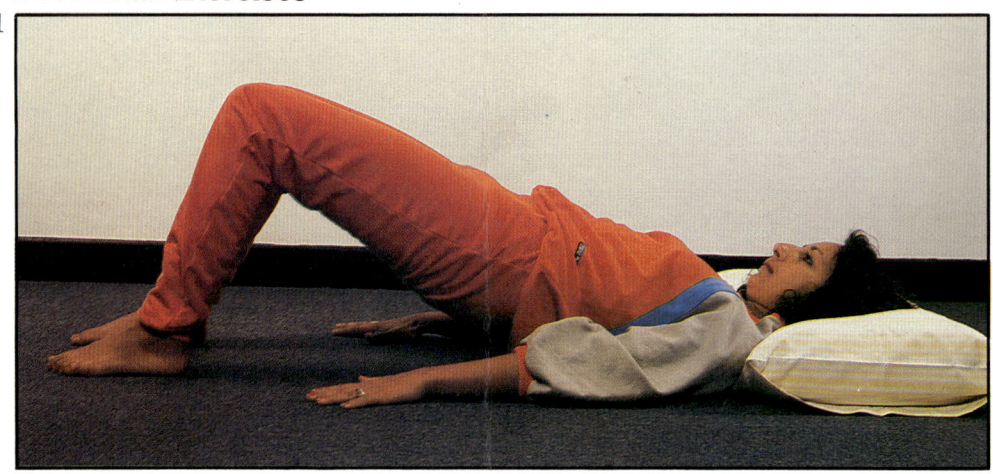

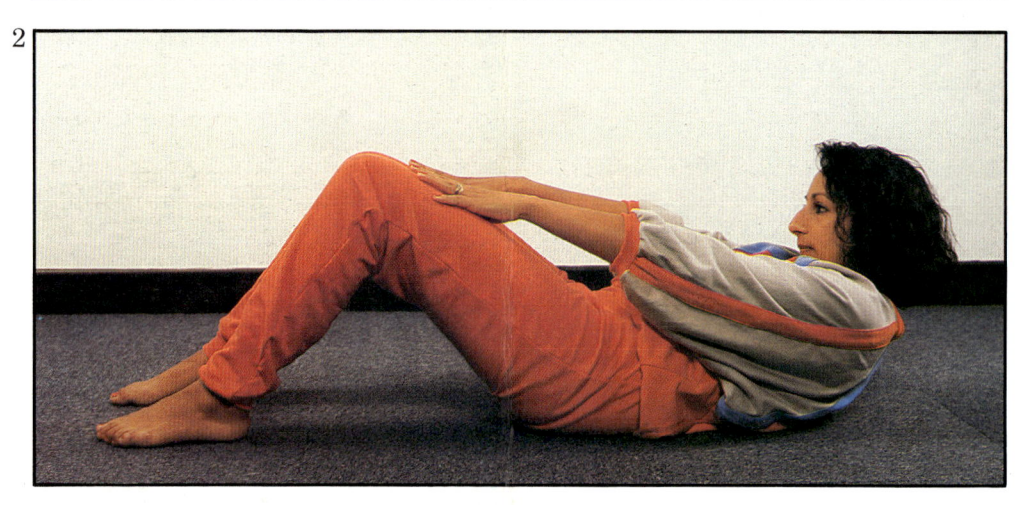

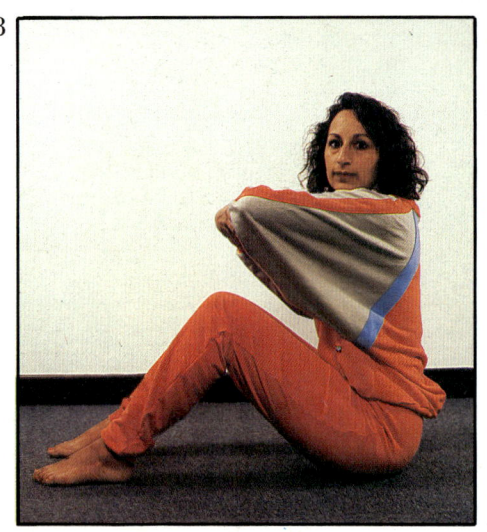

1 Pelvic Floor Toner
Lying on your back, legs bent and feet hip-width apart, gradually tighten pelvic floor muscles and thrust hips up so that knees are in line with shoulders; relax muscles slowly as you lower hips.

2 Tummy Strengtheners
Lie on your back with knees bent, feet apart and hands on thighs. Slowly raising head and shoulders, drop chin and curl up, sliding hands towards knees. Slowly lower body and relax. Repeat 10 times daily.

3 Curl Ups
Try curling up to a sitting position but with arms bent and fingers touching shoulder, then curl down. Repeat 10 times daily.

Exercising with Baby

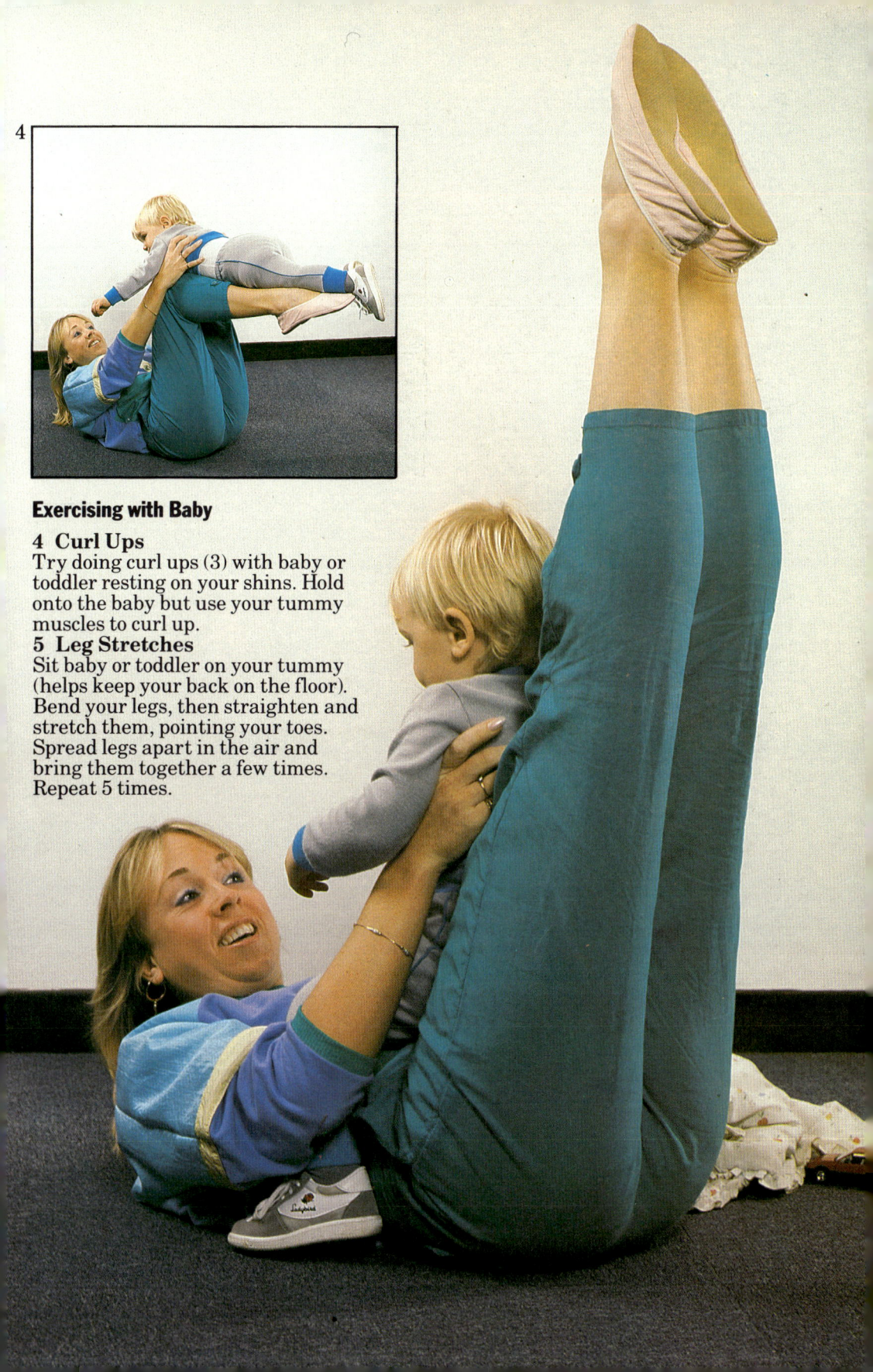

4 Curl Ups
Try doing curl ups (3) with baby or toddler resting on your shins. Hold onto the baby but use your tummy muscles to curl up.

5 Leg Stretches
Sit baby or toddler on your tummy (helps keep your back on the floor). Bend your legs, then straighten and stretch them, pointing your toes. Spread legs apart in the air and bring them together a few times. Repeat 5 times.

MAJOR BODY CHANGES

Development of Pregnancy

Week	
2	Ovulation
3	Conception
4	Period missed; beta-HCG blood pregnancy test positive
5	Perhaps feel as if period about to start; passing urine more often; constipation
6	Nausea am or pm; urine pregnancy test positive
7	May feel dizzy or faint; breasts increase in size and Montgomeray's tubercles appear; feeling very tired; emotionally labile; pregnancy can be confirmed by vaginal examination
8	Increased vaginal discharge; 'go off' certain foods, alcohol and tobacco; may have food cravings; reflexes slower, and clumsy
9	May notice skin changes; gums softening; bra too tight
10	Uterus size of orange
11	Nausea should be lessening; blood volume has increased
12	Uterus has risen out of pelvis; doctor can feel pregnancy; first clinic visit
13	Feeling more active and much less tired
14	Dark line down centre of abdomen
15	All—except very loose clothes, too tight; Cardiac output increased by 20%
16	Pregnancy starts to show
17	May be sweating more
18	Baby may be kicking—felt as fluttering or 'butterflies'
19	Weight gain evident if not before now
20	Uterus pushing up against lungs; navel may protrude; baby increasingly active
21	May get heartburn
22	Baby settling into periods of rest and activity—which are opposed to yours
23	Different parts of baby can be felt; may feel stitch-like pain inside tummy—muscles stretching, pain goes with rest
24	Top of uterus just below navel
25	May notice leg cramps
26	Baby pressing on bladder causing frequency
27	Weight gain at regular rate now until 30 wks
28	Colostrum may leak from breasts
29	Aware of pressure of baby on diaphragm, liver, stomach and gut
30	May develop tingling in fingers (carpal tunnel syndrome*)
31	May become very breathless climbing stairs
32	Increasing tiredness
33	You can distinguish baby's bottom from foot or knee
34	Will be going to antenatal or mothercraft classes
35	May experience quite severe backache—ligaments and muscles of back are relaxing, also baby might be in posterior position
36	Baby's head engages about now: 'lightening' baby settles down in pelvis and makes breathing easier
37	May notice baby hiccupping
38	Baby moving less now (has far less room)
39	Feeling very heavy and weary
40	Term

(* related to weight gain and fluid retention)

MAJOR BODY CHANGES

	If you are accustomed to:			
	Competitive Exercise	**Regular Exercise**	**Pre-conception Exercise**	**Little or no Exercise**
Dos	Continue as before. You should know your own body well and therefore put on the brakes when you feel 'different' to before. Keep up your fluid intake.	Continue as before, but do listen to your body. Drink plenty of fluids. If you want to buy new sports bra, buy 1 or 2 sizes up from the old one.	Keep on slowly and steadily in these 3 months as the baby is settling in. Maintain fitness through gentle stretching, swimming and cycling.	Don't do any straight sit-ups. If you want to cycle, avoid built-up areas and traffic —your reflexes are diminished.
Dont's	Don't train or compete to a point where you are overtired or exhausted. Don't allow your body to overheat.	Make sure you don't do too much. Don't do anything extra just because you're pregnant. Don't allow yourself to overheat, and don't do any straight sit-ups.	Don't do any straight sit-ups. If you want to cycle, avoid built-up areas and traffic——your reflexes are diminished.	Don't do anything strenuous to 'catch up', but don't stop all movement! Don't start cycling now (especially in traffic) unless you are very confident and know how to. Don't do any aerobics.
Dos	Continue, but ease up on mileage or length of workout if necessary. Supplement with walking and swimming. Drink plenty. Start pelvic floor exercises (p. 80).	Continue as before. Do plenty of stretching exercises to maintain suppleness. Start pelvic floor exercises (p. 80).	Keep going gently. Supplement with stretching exercises, walking, swimming, or other non-vigorous sport. Start doing pelvic floor exercises (p. 80).	Get into the habit of doing gently stretching exercises on awakening. Walk, jog, swim, and play some gentle tennis, badminton or golf. Start pelvic floor exercises (p. 80).
Dont's	Don't go in for any serious competition unless well within your reach. Don't lift heavy weights. Don't ski alone in case of falls. Don't cycle unless confident about your new sense of balance.	Don't ski cross-country alone in case of falls. Don't cycle unless confident about your new sense of balance. Don't take up any new jarring sports. Don't lift any heavy weights.	Don't cycle unless confident about your new sense of balance. Don't take up any new jarring sports—even aerobics. Don't lift heavy weights even if previously part of training programme.	Don't take up any new jarring sports like judo, horse-riding or skiing—or even aerobics. Don't lift *any* heavy weights.
Dos	Watch out for injury though—hormone relaxin loosening ligaments and joints making injury much more likely. Continue with pelvic floor exercises.	Take it easy now and watch out for injury. Try doing more swimming and less of the other sports— you can swim up to delivery. Continue with pelvic floor exercises.	Ease right off now if you feel at all tired. Gentle swimming will relax you and keep your muscles in trim. Continue with pelvic floor exercises.	Continue with gentle stretching exercises on waking and try to go swimming at least 3 times per week. Continue with pelvic floor exercises.
Dont's	Don't be afraid to ease off now, and switch to swimming—can swim up until delivery.	Don't take part in any contact sports.	Don't take part in any contact sports. Endeavour to walk 1 mile a day—ie, 15–20 mins brisk pace. Or swim 2–3	Don't *begin* your exercise programme now—except pelvic floor exercises. Make a resolution to begin exercising after delivery, although try to walk a little ($\frac{1}{2}$ mile) every day.

Menopause

Commonly called the change of life, it disappoints many women because life does not change. Certainly the implication is that if it does, it will be for the worse rather than better. Like every physical change since puberty, no one experience is ever the same as anyone else's.

What Happens

The menopause is rather like puberty —but in reverse. It takes place over several years (the climacteric) and may begin as early as 38 years or as late as the mid-50s, though the average age is 51. There is a gradual decline in the functioning of the ovaries with a decrease in the level of oestrogens. In response to this the level of pituitary hormones (gonadotrophins)—especially follicle stimulating hormone (FSH) and luteinising hormone (LH) rises dramatically. This causes a lengthening or shortening of the menstrual cycle in the years up to the menopause, and a variation in the amount of blood lost. Increasingly, also, the cycles become anovular. It is important to remember, however, that the post-menopausal ovary does not stop working altogether, but continues to produce sex hormones for many years.

The Symptoms

Women have probably always had some symptoms at the menopause, but because it means the end of reproductive life, the menopause has been enveloped in as much superstition and myth as menstruation. However, it is wrong to deny that the symptoms at the menopause are real, pretending instead that they are psychological in origin or even, hysterical. In Britain something like 15% of all women have no symptoms but while 85% have anything from slight to severe repercussions, only about 25% have real problems.

Nevertheless, for these women, the menopause can be a miserable time with hot flushes (or flashes) and sweats disturbing sleep, causing insomnia, chronic tiredness and irritability and the hormonal changes affecting the lining of the vagina making intercourse painful, and greatly predisposing to infection. There may also be changes in the lining of the bladder causing pain and frequency and also predisposing to infection.

Treatment: This will depend on the type and severity of the symptoms. But it is important not to underestimate the depressing effect of persistent symptoms even if they are minor. If vaginal dryness and itching are the only problems, then vaginal oestrogen creams may be prescribed together with the suggestion of KY jelly as a lubricant for intercourse. However, for a larger array of symptoms hormonal treatment with oestrogen, progestogen, or a combination of the two might be very effective—although probably not recommended for long term use. There are also some non-hormonal forms of treatment for hot flushes and sweats. No form of drug therapy is ever without risk. This must always be weighed against the benefits and habits or features of lifestyle changed so that the risks are minimised.

Exercise: As the body is going through another of its complex changes, the fitter it is, the better it can cope with the renewed stresses and strains. The value of exercise cannot be emphasised enough, and should be built into a healthy lifestyle at least from the start of the forties. Exercise also helps you relax, keeps you more occupied, stops you nibbling and putting on weight, and helps you sleep more deeply and more tranquilly. Like all the physical changes that a woman goes through, it is again the psychological aspects that need to be boosted and exercise can contribute to this too. It is the positive benefits of sport and exercise, the sense of achievement especially if you set yourself targets—which all help boost your resolve to get through menopause and come out on the other side ready to cash in on a life free from menstruation and contraception problems, still able to enjoy sex to the full and ready to take on new challenges.

Osteoporosis

The added benefit of exercise is to combat osteoporosis, the medical term for brittle bones. You may have noticed that it is older women who break hip and thigh bones quite frequently when they fall over. This is because their bones don't seem to 'hold' calcium as well. However exercise is recognised as a positive benefit. The stretching of the muscles, pulling at tendons on bones puts pressure on those bones, and the bones react to the pressure by becoming more dense. Researchers at the University of North Carolina at Chapel Hill have found that 'Physical activity can significantly reduce the loss of bone that commonly afflicts women as they age'. In the study, conducted among more than 300 women aged 18 to 75 athletic women of all ages had denser bones than those who were inactive. Bone density in active women aged 55 to 75 years was 15 to 20% greater in the spine than in sedentary women of the same age. Since fewer than 20% of the postmenopausal active women took oestrogen supplements, a treatment that is known to slow bone loss, the researchers said, 'hormonal treatment could not account for the differences observed'. The study revealed the special value of exercise that involves gravitational stress. Thus, walking, cycling and tennis were more likely to result in dense bones than swimming. The researchers noted, however, that swimming had other benefits.

Growing Older

The oldest recorded mother is a 57-year-old American but the average age for ceasing sexual activity is 60—not because you have to but because most women feel that you ought to. Tied into this psychological attitude is a whole skein of similar assumptions that 'life is coming to an end' and yet most American and European women have on average another 21 years to live, a quarter of their lives! We are so affected by what we *think* we can do that we end up underestimating our possibilities. Old folk who are still playing golf or writing books or organising charities are regarded as admirable, 'but I'd never be able to do that'...

Latecomers to sport and exercise, where there are less constrictions, less social mores, find that they outstrip their ambitions, let alone live up to them. The *New York Times* reported on a remarkable group of women who took up a seemingly unbeatable challenge and trampled it underfoot:

Tuesday October 12th 1982

You see them in Central Park, along the rivers, anywhere else that runners run. They wear the same colourful racing clothes, the same thick-soled shoes. The major difference is their age: they are over 60, their hair is often gray and, when they run in races, spectators sometimes call out things like 'Come on, Grandma, you can do it.'

But they don't care. As they see it, running is one of the best things that ever happened to them. 'It's a way of life,' said Althea Jureidini, 64, a retired nurse from Brooklyn, who started running at the age of 60. 'It's one thing I can do where I don't feel like an appendage of my husband. I look forward to doing it until I'm 100.' 'I think it's the happiest thing I ever did,' added Evelyn Havens, 66, of Manhattan, who started running four years ago to combat a severe case of arthritis. Since then she has completed 90 races and 7 marathons and 1982 was named 'Senior Woman of the Year' by the New York Road Runners Club. These two are among a growing number of women who are turning to running around retirement age. In many cases, the women had never put on running shoes until they were in their 60s. Some just jog a few blocks a week; others like Jureidini and Havens, are serious competitors. Havens *prefers* races for men and women, such as the New York City Marathon, to those for women only. 'I just love passing guys who are younger,' she said with a smile. 'I like it when they're weaving and staggering and keeling over. It's such a good feeling.'

MAJOR BODY CHANGES

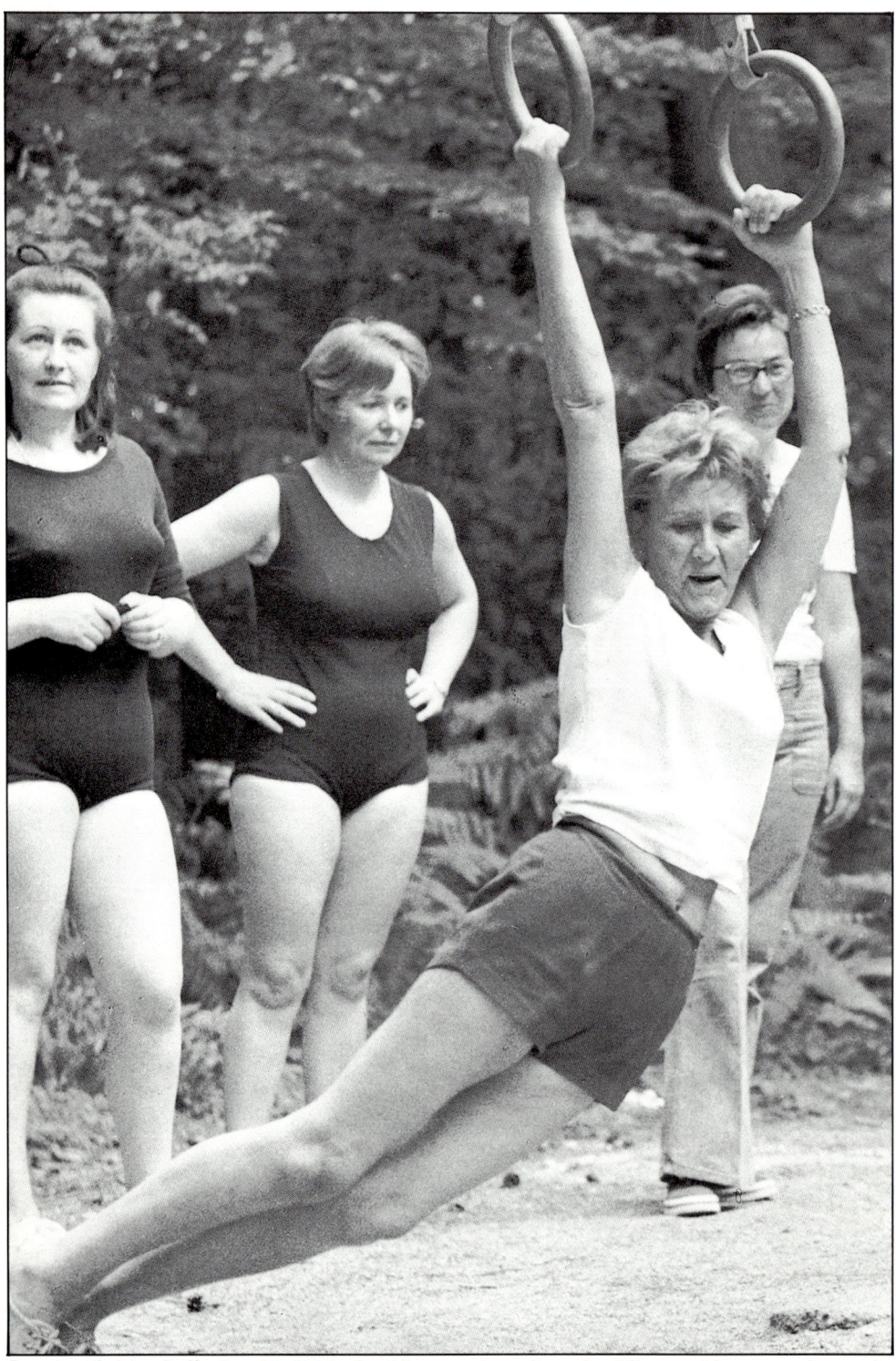

A sense of shared effort and individual achievement can be gained from outdoor exercise such as Parcours, which offers informal training suitable for a wide age range.

For many of these women, running helped fill a void in their lives. Jureidini, whose six daughters are grown, said she was getting 'plain bored' around the house until she started going to a nearby park to watch people run. Eventually she put on track shoes and began to jog. But weak knees forced her to turn to racewalking, a category in which she has since won more than 75 awards. 'The first time I made two miles,' she said, 'I felt like someone had given me $1,000.'

For Adrienne Salamini, 66, a retired nurse from Yonkers, the impetus to start running came four years ago when her oldest son, a runner, gave her a red sweatshirt and sneakers for Mother's Day. She has been so successful that today a room in her house has been reserved for the 170 trophies she has won. And when she walks down the street these days, her husband, Ambrose, tells her to 'slow up, slow up' because she walks so fast. 'You get used to a certain pace,' she explained. 'It's hard to amble anymore.'

They believe in 15 minutes of warm-up and stretching exercises before running and cooling down exercises after running; they eat vitamin-rich food, and they have nearly eliminated red meat from their diets. 'I also take a lot of alfalfa for my arthritis,' said Havens, who runs the office at a vitamin and health food store. Has running helped her arthritis? 'I used to walk with a decided limp, because of arthritis in my feet,' she said. 'Now I no longer limp.'

The women who average about 30 miles a week, said that they viewed running as an excellent way to control weight and appetite. All said they had lost or stabilised their weight and had firmed up flabby flesh after they began running. Perhaps as a result, all look about 15 years younger than they are.

Again, it's never too late to start some sort of exercise and time and time again the body shows what a wonderful machine it is, given the chance. Flabby muscles that have done little or nothing for a whole lifetime perk up when given a gentle workout. And active bodies go hand in hand with active minds, reiterating the Greek saying 'Healthy body, healthy mind', which should shame youngsters who laugh at old folk who go jogging, dancing, keeping busy and having fun.

Exercises for the over-50s need to stimulate the circulation, keep the joints mobile and the muscles, that hold us together, in trim. Instead of trying to keep everything in motion at once, you may need to do a little at a time—working on ankles only, for example, until you are confident that you have the strength and resilience to do something more strenuous. The sociability factor should not be ignored either. One keep-fit class for older folk in England featured two ladies who sat on their exercise bikes for half an hour. They chatted happily throughout the session, even though the pedals never turned! But they had had a good time, made friends and stimulated their brains.

If you want scientific proof that keeping fit also helps to keep you young, you can get a copy of a report published by the Mount Sinai Medical Center at the University of Wisconsin. Doctors there tested veteran runners over a period of ten years and found that those that maintained the same intensity of effort had retained the same aerobic capacity. So the 10% per decade decrease in fitness that doctors acknowledge to be the norm has actually been halted in their case. Ten years of research in the Soviet Union came up with similar results. They found that two 90-minute sessions per week plus walking and/or cross-country skiing not only slowed down older folk's natural decline but even managed to *reverse* it! Blood pressure dropped, lung capacity improved and active people recovered from exertions more quickly than inactive older people.

Whereas most people over 50 think of doing a little *less* in deference to their age, they should be thinking of doing something *more* because exercise creates more energy rather than 'using up' what you have. Marion Irvine was an inspiration to older women when she qualified for the US Olympic trials at the age of 54. Her event? The marathon! What's more she only took up distance running at the age of 48—and she is a nun. Her personal best was 2 hours 50 minutes.

Nutrition and Diet

The effect of nutrition and diet in our lives is greatly underestimated. It may be said that in western society, we are overfed but undernourished. The typical diet is far from balanced; we eat too much of many things — sugar in tea and coffee, quick snacks as 'fillers' with little nutritional value — and hope to remedy the situation by topping up with vitamin pills and mineral supplements. Because what and how we eat directly reflects our lifestyles, the move to a healthier diet requires a new outlook on life. A re-evaluation of dietary needs is the natural complement to regular exercise and increasing vigour.

Back to Basics

What's in Food?

The basic constituents of food are proteins, fats, carbohydrates, and water. They serve to keep the body in working order by building and maintaining cells and tissues, supplying energy for all the metabolic processes—including keeping you warm—and allowing for the transport of hormones and inter-cell messages in solution.

The body also needs the micro-nutrients: vitamins, minerals, and trace elements. These are involved in the metabolism of proteins, fats and carbohydrates, help promote tissue structure and function, catalyse biochemical reactions, and are vital for the formation of blood cells, muscles and bones. Some of these the body can make for itself, but most must be supplied from food.

Your Nutritional Requirements: These vary throughout your life, depending on physiological changes in your body—such as growth in childhood and during pregnancy, your state of health or ill health and level of activity. They also, though to a lesser extent, depend on your lifestyle habits: tea, coffee, tobacco, and alcohol all rob your body of vitamins, just as over-cooking vegetables, leaving milk bottles on doorsteps exposed to sunlight, and cooking in copper pots destroys some vitamins. However, the chart on p. 102 outlines all your basic nutritional requirements and lists the richest food sources in descending order. There are also comments on function, increased needs, and risks of toxicity.

Calories

The calorie is a unit of heat which is used to describe the amount of energy available from food. All food has the potential to supply energy—sometimes instantly (sugar), sometimes gradually (starches and complex carbohydrates), and sometimes indirectly (excess protein)—and therefore contains calories. Excess food—energy—is stored in the liver and muscles as

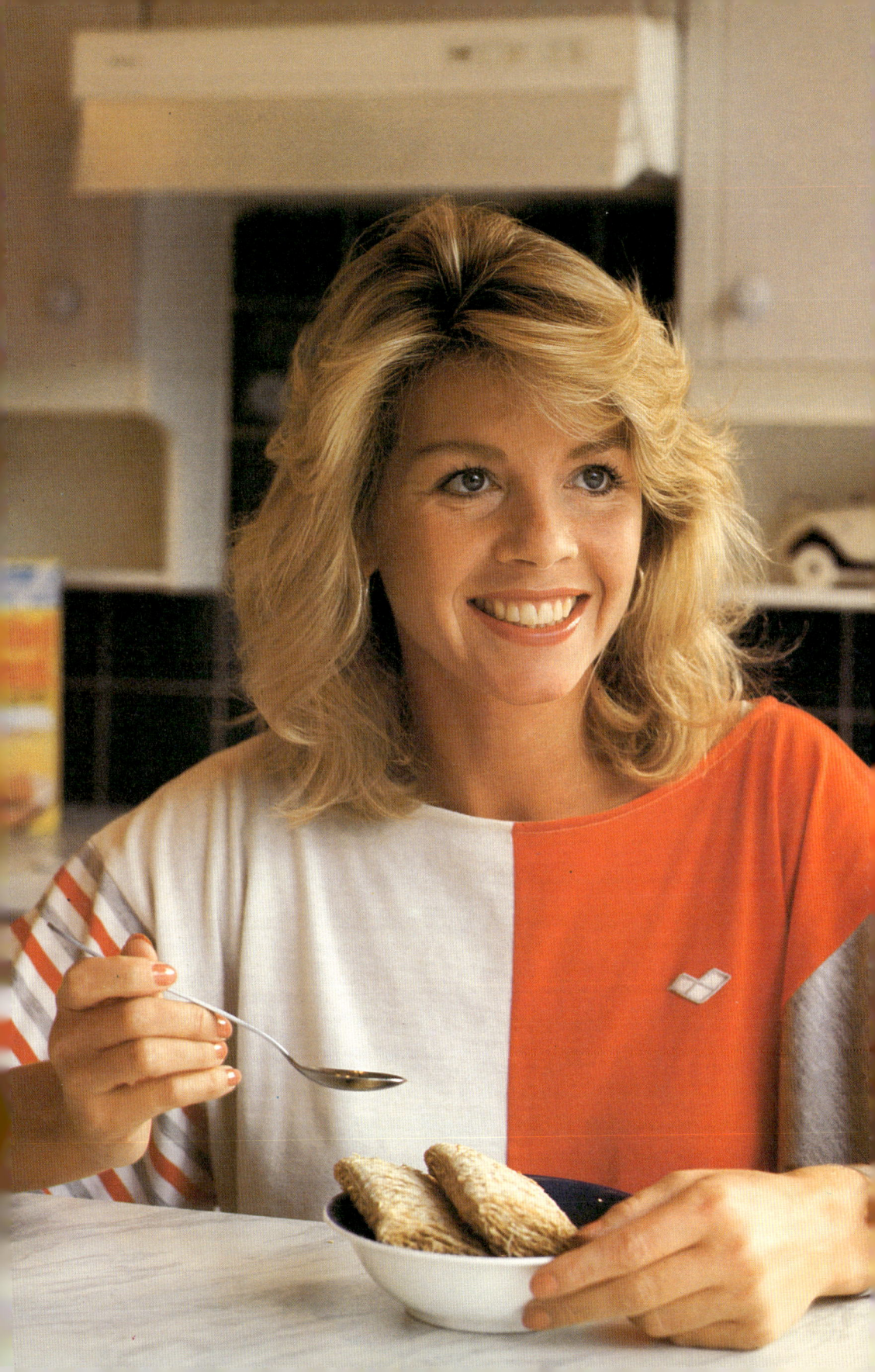

glycogen, and under the skin as fat. (This is a form of adaptation which harks back to the days of primitive man when it was necessary to survive lean periods, when no food was available for days or weeks, by drawing on fat reserves for energy.) Although this survival mechanism persists and is largely in evidence, it is, in the West, superfluous as we are surrounded by—and consume—an overabundance of food.

Your Basic Energy Requirement: This depends on age, size, metabolic rate and level of activity, so there is no absolute, ideal calorie count. However, you can gain a rough guide to the amount of food energy you need to take in by multiplying your weight in pounds by 15 (or weight in kilograms by 33). The resulting figure is the number of calories needed daily to maintain your current weight. Using the same method of calculation, you can also work out the number needed to maintain your ideal, rather than actual, weight. The difference between the two figures represents the adjustment you should make to daily calorie intake in order to achieve your ideal weight-by how many calories you should decrease or increase your food intake in order to lose or gain weight.

Adjusting the Balance

Just as important as the quantity of food—ie, energy or calories, is the quality. A diet consisting solely of sugar, might supply all the energy your body needs, but would, very quickly, make you ill as you are not providing your body with all the other nutrients it needs.

The problem at present is that we tend to eat too much protein, too much saturated fat (SAFA) and simple carbohydrates like sugar. As the table on p. 97 shows, we need to reduce our overall consumption of protein and SAFA—particularly where they overlap: milk, cheese, butter, meat—and eat more vegetable proteins, polyunsaturated fats, and drastically cut down on sugar and refined carbohydrates, replacing them with unrefined and complex carbohydrates in the form of starches and dietary fibre.

Breakfast

If there's one meal that is ignored nowadays, it is breakfast. Grab a cup of coffee and run is how many of us start our day, putting ourselves under stress straight away. It is easy enough, and healthy too, to have a bowl of muesli in the morning. This ensures a good supply of carbohydrates as well as the fibre your digestive system needs. Otherwise, from the time you go to bed to your next 'reasonable' meal—a sandwich at lunch—could well be over 12 hours. It's no wonder then that we put sugar into coffee and tea and reach for chocolate mid-morning. It makes far more nutritional sense to eat breakfast with a day's work ahead, than to starve and wait for a big meal in the evening when your metabolism is slowing down in readiness for 7 or 8 hours sleep.

If you can't face eating first thing but then find that you're famished by 10 or 11 o'clock, try getting up earlier to give your body time to wake up. Do some stretching exercises, go for a walk or jog, get some of the household chores you normally leave until the evening, out of the way. You'll feel fresher and feel you've achieved something. You will also have an appetite for breakfast and be better prepared to start the day.

A Good Start

- Sugar-free or home-made muesli with skimmed milk. (Soak the muesli overnight in milk or apple juice to make it more digestible, if you wish)
- Natural, live yoghurt with or without fresh or dried fruit
- A few pieces of dried fruit and a handful of nuts or seeds
- Porridge
- Boiled egg with wholemeal toast
- Wholemeal toast spread very lightly with butter, polyunsaturated margarine, or a low-fat spread, and low-sugar marmalade or jam
- Fresh fruit—eating an orange (rather than just drinking the juice) gives you fibre as well as vitamin C
- Sugar-free cereal with skimmed milk

Cholesterol

Cholesterol is a vitally important part of every cell in the body. It is also a precursor to many steroid hormones. The main source of cholesterol in the diet is from saturated animal fats. Excess cholesterol accumulates as fatty streaks in the lining of the major arteries and ultimately becomes an obstruction to blood flow.

In the young woman, the female sex hormone oestrogen actively removes cholesterol from the peripheral tissues to the liver via the gall bladder. This is the reason why pre-menopausal women (not on the Pill) are generally protected from coronary heart disease (CHD). (It also explains, paradoxically, the risks of gall bladder disease in this group.) Once women reach the menopause, their oestrogen levels drop and statistics show a correspondingly sharp increase in coronary heart disease in women over 50. But although it looks as though oestrogen protects against CHD, it is in fact only the naturally produced (endogenous) hormone which does this —as researchers discovered, with tragic results, when they gave oestrogen to men and actually *precipitated* deaths from CHD.

Whole milk is a rich source of both cholesterol and oestrogen, so you should switch to skimmed milk and limit your intake of saturated fats (SAFA). If you do this, you will be limiting your intake of cholesterol automatically—although there are some dietary items which are high sources of cholesterol which may not be obvious (see table).

Hunger vs Appetite

There is a world of difference between being hungry for food and having an appetite for something. The sensation of hunger is brought about by a decrease in the blood glucose concentration and is accompanied by contractions of the stomach and feeling tense and restless. Appetite, on the other hand, is influenced by many situations: conditioning to expect food at certain times, the sight, smell or even the thought of food. While a little bit of what you fancy may do you good, in the long run it makes for overweight if we tend to eat when we're not really hungry.

Hunger and Exercise

Inactivity increases appetite. Appetite is controlled by the 'appestat' at the base of the brain. When there is little physical activity, this regulatory mechanism is upset and appetite increases. Meanwhile, even a little exercise will raise the blood glucose and fight off a feeling of hunger. It is interesting to remind ourselves mid-morning when glucose levels are reduced, and we are tempted to have another cup of sugary coffee, that children in schools are emptied out onto the playgrounds at this time to run around and so raise their blood glucose and perk themselves up *that* way.

Sources of Cholesterol

Low	Medium	High
All fruit and vegetables; polyunsaturated margarines, corn, safflower and sunflower seed oils, skimmed milk, low-fat yoghurt, cottage cheese, chicken, turkey, white fish, lobster, egg white, most nuts, flour, bread, pasta, breakfast cereals.	Avocado, bacon, beef, hard cheese, coffee creamers, eggs, lamb, ham, pork, tinned meat, tinned fish, oily fish, olives, olive oil.	Butter, hard margarine, whole milk, cream, lard, ice cream, sour cream, cream cheese, chocolate, cashew nuts, tongue, offal, most shellfish, cod's roe, manufactured baked goods.

Tips on Cooking, Buying and Eating Food

- Eat food raw as much as possible
- Buy food as close to its original form as possible – eg, fresh fish rather than fish cakes
- Avoid sweetened drinks. Buy fruit juice and dilute with water
- Try herb teas (cut out sugar and milk)
- Replace whole milk with semi-skimmed, skimmed or soya milk
- Don't overcook vegetables or add salt or soda bicarbonate to cooking water
- Don't have second helpings
- Replace sugary deserts with fresh or stewed fruit or live natural yoghurt and fruit
- Live yoghurt is the only form of yoghurt that has any health or nutritional benefit
- The moment you feel full, stop eating – regardless of how much is left on your plate
- Don't over-eat when you feel stressed or anxious
- Snack on fresh fruit rather than chocolate or biscuits

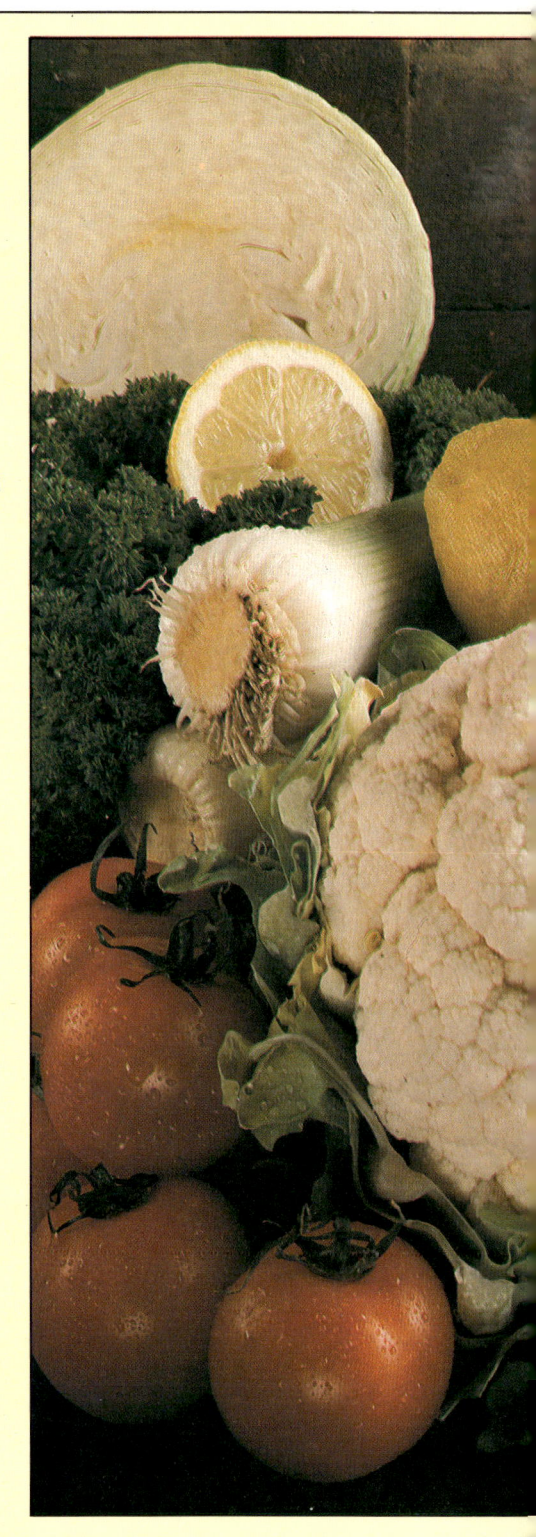

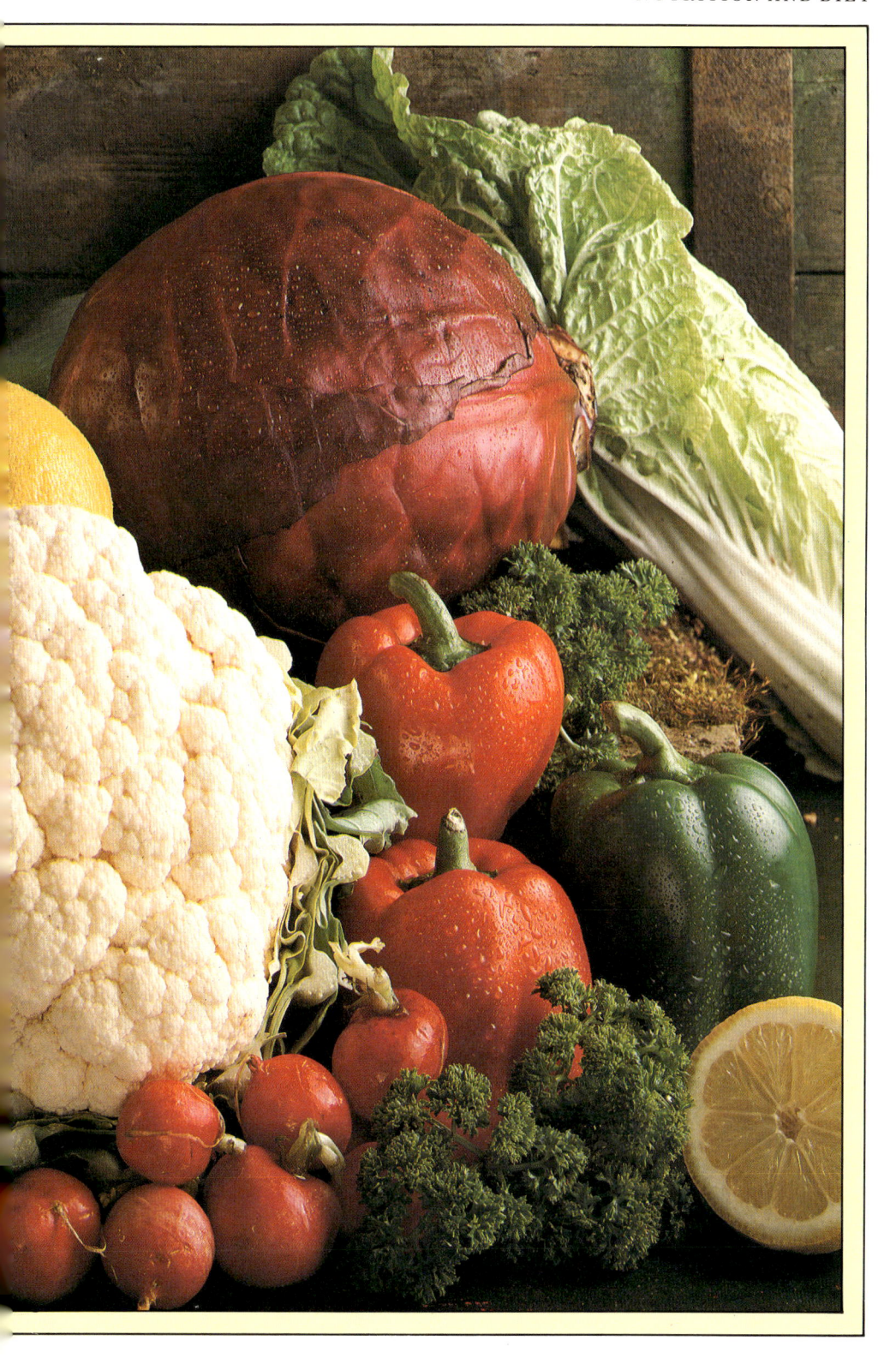

NUTRITION AND DIET

Guidelines for Healthy Eating

Faulty eating habits and acquired tastes are difficult to change, so dietary modifications are best introduced gradually if you are to succeed in re-educating your and your family's tastes.

Proteins

Although protein is part and parcel of the fabric of our bodies and therefore essential for health, we tend to eat twice as much as we actually need. Cut down on meat, whole milk, cheese and butter, and replace with fish, skimmed or semi-skimmed milk, cereals and pulses (peas, lentils and beans). Pulses have a negligible fat content, are very nutritious, cheap, and very filling. Their only drawback is that they must be soaked overnight before cooking. While it doesn't mean you have to become a vegetarian, there are plenty of good vegetarian and ethnic cook books on the market with delicious recipes for inspirational meals.

Fats

Look at the table on p. 98 and cut right back on saturated animal fats: meat, dairy products etc. These are rich sources of cholesterol. Replace them with polyunsaturated fats (PUFA), including fish oils which have a beneficial effect on the circulatory system.

Carbohydrates

Unrefined and complex carbohydrates should become the mainstay of your diet.

Sugar: Basically, we do not need carbohydrate in this form. It rots teeth, makes you susceptible to diabetes and upsets blood glucose levels so that you may feel washed out but crave for more. Gradually learn to cut sugar right out of your diet—whether white or brown—and don't be fooled into thinking that honey is anything other than sugar. For cooking, try using blackstrap molasses to impart sweetness; it contains some minerals. Avoid rewarding children with sweets or chocolate. This is not only bad for the teeth but gives them a 'sweet tooth' that will not stand them in good stead in the years ahead.

Read labels when shopping: sugar is added to just about everything—except disinfectant! Be wary of breakfast cereals, as most contain sugar. Home-made muesli is fun to mix (if you don't like raisins you can leave them out and not feel you're wasting a small fortune by leaving them at the side of your cereal bowl) and in the long run, cheaper than any commercial variety or cereal.

Starch: Potatoes are not fattening! It is only when you start to fry them or smother them in butter that you're piling on excess calories. Eat *more* potatoes (and their skins) and more fruit and vegetables. They're filling, contain fibre for your digestive system and supply your body with energy in 'sustained release' form.

Complex: Eat more fibrous food: wholemeal and grain breads, raw fruit and vegetables, nuts, seeds, dried fruit, peas, beans etc. They speed up the transit time of wastes in the bowel and so reduce the accumulation of toxins which could predispose to disease. Fibre-rich diets have been shown to be very beneficial for many conditions ranging from Crohn's disease to diabetes. Add bran to soups and stews and when baking, to cakes and bread. This is preferable to merely sprinkling bran on your cereals. When first changing to a high-fibre diet you may get a bloated tummy and gas pains, which will settle as your body adjusts.

Additives

Read the label! Be wary of listed additives and words like 'colour', 'flavour' etc. These are added to foods to make them look more appetising and to prolong shelf-life. However, they have been implicated in a host of 'allergic' conditions as well as industrial dermatitis, (in workers handling these chemicals) gastritis, colitis, arthritis, migraine and hyperactivity in children.

Salt

Although we consist of 8 pints of salted water and many biochemical reactions take place with salt (sodium) in the

NUTRITION AND DIET

Healthy Eating

	PROTEIN	FAT	CARBOHYDRATE
FUNCTION	Essential constituents of body: form and maintain muscles, tissues, organs etc. Protein is broken down into amino acids which are then re-arranged to make proteins as required. Excess can be converted into glucose.	Provides energy, insulation, vitamins A, D, E, K, and essential fatty acids. Excess stored as fatty tissue. 1. SAFA: Saturated fats. 2. MUFA: Mono-unsaturated fats. 3. PUFA: Polyunsaturated fats.	Provides energy in the form of glucose for all metabolic processes stored in liver and muscles. Excess is converted into fat. 1. SUGAR: Rapid energy supply, but sudden, high blood-sugar triggers insulin release to bring this back down to 'normal'. This drop in blood-sugar leads to renewed hunger pangs and craving for more sugar. Exception is fructose which is metabolised slowly. 2. STARCH: Gradual but steady energy source. 3. COMPLEX: Poor energy source; undigested.
FOOD EXAMPLES	Meat, fish, eggs, cheese, nuts, pulses, cereals, bread.	SAFA: Meat, milk, cheese, butter, cream. MUFA: Fish, poultry, ground nut and olive oils. PUFA: Fish, fish oils, plant foods, safflower oil.	SUCROSE: All forms of sugarbeet and cane. GLUCOSE: Honey, all carbohydrate once broken down. FRUCTOSE: Fruit, fruit juices, honey. LACTOSE: Milk. All cereals, vegetables, and fruit. CELLULOSE: Vegetables. PECTIN: Fruit. BRAN: Cereals.

PERCENTAGE AVERAGE DAILY CALORIE INTAKE

CURRENT	PROTEIN 20%	FAT 40%	CARBOHYDRATE 40%
IDEAL	PROTEIN 11%	FAT 30%	CARBOHYDRATE 59%

body, we don't *need* to add any to our food. Read labels. Like sugar, salt is added to very many things. All flavour enhancers contain salt in some form. And you do not need extra salt when exercising!

Caffeine
This is a stimulant and in excess can lead to effects ranging from headache and irritability to insomnia and palpitations. Count the number of cups of tea, coffee, cola and cocoa drinks you consume each day and cut by half. Try cereal or dandelion beverages instead, and herb teas. These are a new but rapidly acquired taste and don't need milk (or sugar!). If you're thirsty, drink tap or mineral water or diluted, no added-sugar, fruit juices.

Alcohol
Alcohol contains as many calories as fat and actively interferes with the absorption of some vitamins and essential fatty acids. Cut out all spirits and be very moderate with wine and beer.

NUTRITION AND DIET

Food Alternatives

Fat

CUT DOWN ON	ALTERNATIVE
Beef, lamb, pork, pies, sausages, hamburgers, bacon etc. Eat red meat once a day at the most, but preferably only 3 times a week.	Chicken, turkey, rabbit, veal, fish (but avoid poultry skin)
Chips, French fries	Baked potatoes
Frying	Grilling (then 'dry off' fat in paper towel)
Lard, shortening, vegetable oil in hard 'blocks'	Sunflower, soya, corn oils; peanut, olive, walnut oils (more expensive)
Butter, cream, ice cream, cream cheese	Margarine (soft tub type, high in polyunsaturates), yogurt-based ice cream, cottage cheese
Whole milk	Skimmed, semi-skimmed, or low fat milk (except for children)
Store-bought biscuits, cookies, cakes	Home-made
High-fat cheese: Cheddar, Parmesan, Stilton, Gorgonzola, processed cheeses	Low-fat: Ricotta, cottage cheese, quark Medium-fat: Edam, Gouda, Brie, Camembert, Jarlsburg

Sugar

CUT DOWN ON	ALTERNATIVE
Sweets, candies, chocolate bars	Fresh fruit; dried fruit and nuts
Canned and bottled goods like spaghetti, ketchup, soups	Sugar-free commercial products (even canned fruit in natural juice)
Cakes, cookies etc, bought in shops	Home-made—using only half recommended amount of sugar or use blackstrap molasses; dried fruit and nut bars (these contain quite a lot of sugar, but bound up with complex carbohydrates)
Cola-type drinks, 'soft' drinks	Diet version, or fruit juices (with no added sugar) diluted with tap or mineral water
Breakfast cereals with added sugar (most)	Low or no sugar varieties; muesli (home-made)
Jellies, jams, spreads	Use low-sugar alternatives; cut thicker slice of bread so you eat only one portion of 'spread' to double portion of bread
Sugar in tea, coffee	Gradually wean yourself off, then go without. Cereal beverages ('Barley Cup'), herbal teas
Sugar on desserts	Spices

Vitamins and Minerals

The three basic features of vitamins and minerals are:

- They are essential for the working of fundamental body processes
- They cannot be made by the body and must therefore be regularly obtained from food. (Vitamins A, D, E, K are fat-soluble and may be stored in fatty tissue in the body. B-Complex vitamins and Vitamin C are water-soluble. They cannot be stored and any excess is lost in the urine)
- They are required in only minute amounts (hundredths or thousandths of a gram)

The metabolism of vitamins and minerals by the body is very complex and many factors can increase or decrease your body's use of these nutrients. For example, cooking and food processing can cause vitamin and mineral loss from food, while less obviously, there may be certain substances within a food which prevent the active absorption of a vitamin. Spinach, for example, has always been thought to be a good source of iron, but on closer inspection, an enzyme in spinach (oxalic acid) interacts with the iron making most of it unavailable to the body. The absorption of iron is increased in the presence of vitamin C and decreased by tannin—as is found in tea. Perhaps equally complicated is the fact that certain foods increase your body's needs for certain vitamins or minerals. A diet rich in carbohydrate for example, necessitates more thiamin (vitamin B_1), while the consumption of alcohol increases your needs for all the B vitamins. Meanwhile, an inactive lifestyle can cause the mobilisation of calcium from its storage in the bones leading to osteoporosis.

Given all these interfering factors it may seem that vitamin and mineral supplements are the surest way of getting what your body needs. But this isn't true. The metabolism of vitamins and minerals *is* complex and some of the problems encountered with absorption from food can also occur with supplements. Taking large doses of zinc, for example, can precipitate copper deficiency. In fact, the taking of vitamins and minerals in this way is analogous to the taking of drugs and should therefore be subject to the same precautions (preparation, dose, interaction, excretion, toxicity). However, people who should consider supplements are those whose diet is restricted for any reason. Vegans for example, who eat no animal products are susceptible to vitamin B_{12} deficiency unless they take supplements, as B_{12} is not found in plant foods.

The most sensible and effective approach to vitamins and minerals is to

Keeping the Goodness In

VITAMINS	CAUSE OF DESTRUCTION OR LOSS
A	High temperature when oxygen present
B_1 (Thiamin)	Exposure to heat above cooking temperature
B_2 (Riboflavin)	Light—eg, milk bottle on doorstep or in glass pitcher in sunny kitchen
	Alkali—eg, baking soda
	Alcohol—soluble
B_6 (Pyridoxine)	Cooking water losses—water-soluble; alcohol-soluble
B_{12} (Cyanocobalamin)	Unstable in hot acid or alkaline solutions
	Cooking water losses, and loss from drip from meat. Alcohol-soluble.
C (Ascorbic acid)	Air—easily destroyed by oxidation: Cook vegetables with saucepan lid on.
	Enzyme released on cutting fruit and vegetables. Vitamin loss can be halted by immediate blanching or delaying food preparation.
	Cooking water losses as water-soluble.
	Copper pans
Folic Acid (Folate/Folacin)	Substantial cooking losses
	Losses when food stored at room temperature
Minerals	Cooking losses

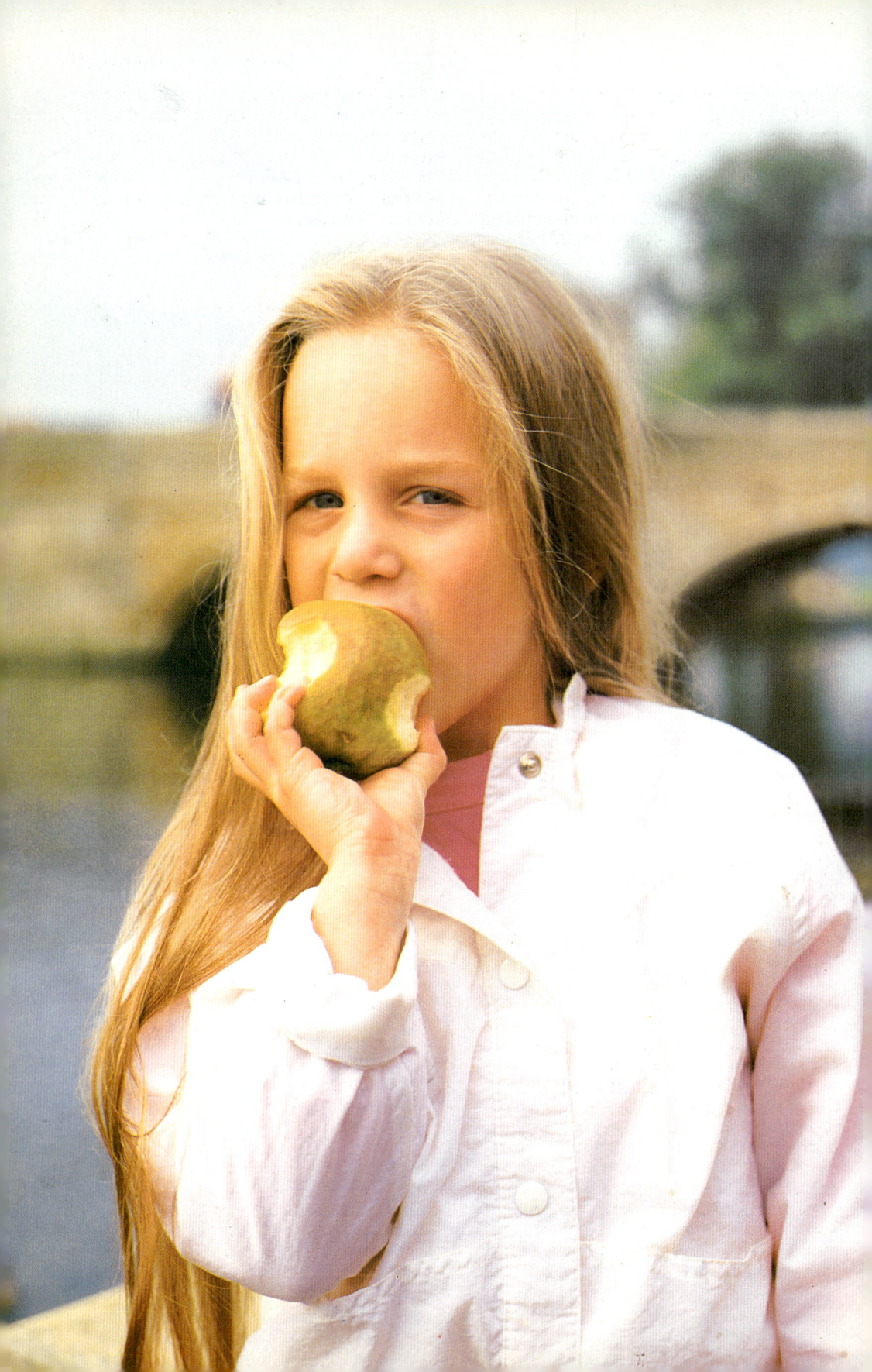

be far more discerning about the kind and quality of food you eat. Generally, the more raw foods you eat the greater will be your intake of vitamins and minerals. Obviously this isn't always practicable, but you can be careful about your preparation and cooking techniques. The table (see p.99) shows vitamin losses which are everyday occurrences and preventable.

Eating and Exercise

Exercise is an important regulator of appetite allowing for the proper working of the 'appestat'. During your work out you are using up available glucose in your blood (usually for the first 20 minutes), thereafter you will begin using your glycogen stores. Exercise also enables you to let off steam, release tension and alleviate boredom which might otherwise create a psychological need to overeat.

Exercise also increases your metabolic rate. This increases while you are exercising (as you expend more energy), but even once you've stopped, the oxidative recovery process continues working. This can have a cumulative effect on increasing your metabolic rate if you work out for 30 minutes or more every day.

As you become fitter you will notice that your taste for food changes: you shun some, and embrace others—usually the more 'healthy' ones. Very often, there is a physiological reason for this.

Metabolism

Your basic metabolism is the absolute minimum amount of energy required to keep your body ticking over. It is highest at birth and during childhood and gradually decreases as you get older which might be one reason why you find that you put on weight even though your calorie intake has not changed. It is related to sex (men have a higher metabolic rate than women), state of health and activity level. Severe cutbacks in calorie intake only serve to slow your metabolic rate down. Weight loss will be faster if a higher metabolism is maintained during exercise.

Calories: If you only do half an hour a day of exercise, you shouldn't need any extra calories. Above that, however, multiply your *bodyweight* in *pounds* (lbs) × 4, and in kilograms (kg) × 8, to get the answer in *Calories required per hour of exercise*.

Diabetes

Diabetes is a lack of, or insufficient insulin, a hormone which keeps the level of sugar in the blood within a fairly narrow range. Diabetics can participate in all sports but may need to adjust their medication or diet if prolonged or exhausting exercise is undertaken.

The most severe diabetics require injections of insulin to control their illness. Any activity which increases the energy requirements—ie, exercise or sport—will, for the insulin-dependent diabetic, mean using less insulin before the exercise period. Or, if the exercise is unplanned or the timing unpredictable, extra carbohydrate should be taken to prevent going 'hypo' (hypoglycaemic: when the blood sugar falls below normal levels). If a diabetic—or a non-diabetic who has so exhausted herself that blood sugar reserves have been depleted—becomes hypoglycaemic, she becomes sweaty, lose concentration, become confused, may become aggressive and can fall unconscious. For this reason, diabetics should wear an identifying bracelet or medallion so that if they do become unconscious care can be undertaken promptly. Initial symptoms can be counteracted with glucose or other carbohydrate but if unconsciousness develops, an injection of glucose is required.

Non-insulin dependent diabetics have milder diabetes and require either tablets to control their blood sugar or a restricted carbohydrate diet to prevent their blood sugar from rising too high since this has harmful effects on blood vessels and other organs. These diabetics are often overweight, but by modifying their diet and introducing exercise, weight loss can ensue and this can improve the control of the diabetes as can exercise alone in the non-overweight diabetic.

Richest food sources in descending order per 100g

Protein (g)	Peanuts & sunflower seeds, 28; Cheddar cheese 25; Almonds 21; Meat 18; Fish 18; Eggs 12; Wholemeal bread 8; Pulses 5; Milk 3.
Fat (g)	PUFA: Vegetable oils 99; Soft margarine 81; Nuts 49; Chicken 17; Fish 0·7. SAFA: Lard 99; Butter 82; Bacon 40; Cheddar cheese 33; Beef 22; Ice cream 8; Milk 4.
Carbohydrate (CHO) (g)	Sugar 100; Honey 80; Cereal grains & Pasta 70–80; Jam 70; Raisins 65; Bread 45; Dried fruit 30–50; Fresh fruit 15; Potatoes 20–40; Cashew nuts 28; Vegetables 2–20; Peanuts 9.
Fibre (g)	Wheat bran 45; All-bran 27; Figs & Apricots (dried) 20; Almonds 14; Jacket potatoes 12; Wholemeal bread 9; Peanuts 8; Cereal grains 7; White bread 3.
Vitamin A (Retinol) (mcg)	Spinach 1000; Margarine 900; Butter 750; Cheese 385; Eggs 140; Liver 18; Cod Liver Oil 18.
Vitamin B_1 (Thiamin) (mg)	Brewer's yeast 15; Yeast extract 3; Brown rise 3; Wheatgerm 2; Brazil nuts 1; Pecans 1; Oats 0·5; Wholemeal bread 0·2.
Vitamin B_2 (Riboflavin) (mg)	Yeast extract 6; Liver 3; Kidney 2; Cheddar cheese 0·5; Eggs 0·5; Milk 0·2.
Nicotinic Acid (Niacin) (mg)	Peanuts 21; Liver 18; Peanut butter 15; Tuna fish 12; Pork 9; Beef 8; Plaice 6; Eggs 4; Bread 3; Lentils 2.
Vitamin B_6 (mg) (Pyridoxine)	Yeast 4; Mackerel 8; Chicken, Pork Plaice, Tuna 0·4; Beef 3; Eggs 0·1; Milk, Bananas, Peanuts, Wholemeal bread 0·1.
Folic Acid (Folacin) (mcg)	Endive 330; Lamb liver 220; Spinach 140; Broccoli 130; Peanuts 110; Walnuts 66; Oranges 37.
Vitamin B_{12} (Cyanocobalamin) (mcg)	Liver (ox) 110; (lamb) 84; Kidney 55; Sardines 28; Pilchards 12; Rabbit 10; Beef, Lamb, Turkey, White Fish 2; Eggs 1·7; Marmite 0·5.
Vitamin C (Ascorbic acid) (mg)	Acerola juice 1200; Blackcurrants (raw) 200; (stewed) 150; Green pepper 127; Strawberries 60; Oranges, Lemons, 50; Grapefruit 40; Brussels sprouts (ckd) 40; Tomatoes 20; Potatoes 10–30; Apples 5; Dried fruit 0.
Vitamin D (Cholecalciferol) (mcg)	Cod liver oil 210; Kippers 25; Herring 22; Mackerel 17; Margarine 8; Tuna fish 6; Eggs 2; Dairy foods contain little.
Vitamin E (Tocopherol) (mg)	Wheatgerm 11; Peanuts 8; Olive oil 5; Muesli 3; Butter 2; Eggs 1·6; Wholemeal flour 1; Cheese 0·8.
Calcium (Ca) (mg)	Cheddar cheese 800; Sardines 550; Camembert 380; Figs (dried) 280; Watercress 220; Milk chocolate 220; Soya flour 210; Yoghurt 170; Molasses 165; Milk 120; Bread 100; Wholemeal bread 23.
Phosphorous (Ph) (mg)	Cheddar cheese 520; Eggs 220; Chicken 200; Cod 170; Beef 160; Yoghurt 140; Note that phosphorus contained in cereals, nuts and pulses cannot be retained by the body.
Magnesium (Mg) (mg)	Winkles 360; Soya flour 240; Shrimps 110; Chocolate 100; Dates 59; Whitebait 50; Bananas 42; Raisins 42.
Iron (Fe) (mg)	Liver 21; Molasses 11; Soya flour 7; Mussels 6; Kidney 5; Apricots (dried) 4; Sardines 3; Beef 2·7; Plain chocolate 2·4; Red wine 1; Note that iron contained in pulses, dark green vegetables and nuts cannot be retained by the body.
Zinc (Zn) (mg)	Lobster 8; Beef 4·3; Lamb 4; Cheddar 4; Sardines 3; Oatmeal 3; Peanuts 3; Eggs 1·5.
Iodine (I) (mcg)	Sea fish; Seaweed; Iodised Salt. Sources yield variable amounts.

NUTRITION AND DIET

Recommended daily intake for women of all ages

1–3	4–6	7–10	11–14	15–18	19–22	23–50	51+	Preg'y	Breast-feeding
30	37	44	53	53	54	54	47	60	69
65	75	93	85	70	70	67	60	80	92
149	219	347	304	314	313	296	268	360	411
10	13	15	18	20	30	35	35	35–40	40
400	300	700	800	800	800	800	800	1000	1400
0·7	0·9	1·2	1·1	1·1	1·1	1·0	1·0	1·4	1·5
0·8	1·0	1·4	1·3	1·3	1·3	1·2	1·2	1·5	1·8
9	11	16	15	14	14	13	13	18	20
0·9	1·3	1·6	1·8	2·0	2·0	2·0	2·0	2·6	2·5
100	200	300	400	400	400	400	400	800	500
2·0	2·5	3·0	3·0	3·0	3·0	3·0	3·0	4·0	4·0
20	45	45	50	60	60	60	60	80	100
10	10	10	10	10	7·5	5	5	12	15
5	6	7	8	8	8	8	8	10	11
800	800	800	1200	1200	800	800	800	1200	1200
800	800	800	1200	1200	800	800	800	1200	1200
150	200	250	300	300	300	300	300	450	450
7	10	10	12	12	12	12	10	13 UK 30 US	15 UK 60 US
10	10	10	15	15	15	15	15	20	30
70	90	120	150	150	150	150	150	175	200

Stress and Addiction

When stress is handled effectively it is a source of motivation — a positive force encouraging us to overcome obstacles and achieve our ambitions and goals. When stress gets the upper hand, however, it masks our abilities and the anxiety and tension can become overwhelming. It is tempting to combat the stress with short-term solutions — alcohol, tobacco, drugs or food — and gradually these become negative addictions seemingly impossible to break. Exercise is a valuable weapon in fighting such cycles of self-destructive behaviour. You cannot eliminate stress from your life, but you can learn to make it work for you.

Stress

Sudden, alarming events which elicit the instinctual 'flight or fight' reaction are not an everyday occurrence. What is much more likely is repeated low-grade threatening situations which gradually cause a build-up of undischarged anxiety and tension, leading to a feeling of physical rigidity and powerlessness in response to overwhelming internal pressure.

This is stress, and it is a vital early warning system. The familiar feelings raised by stress are a deliberate attempt to make us aware of—and preferably confront—those situations which threaten our physical and mental health, self-esteem and happiness.

If stress is the biochemical and psychological consequence of undischarged anxiety and tension and pent-up adrenalin charge, then to ignore the symptoms which result is to invite both physical and mental ill-health.

Coping with Stress

There is no way of avoiding all stressful situations (without some form of stress the human race would die out), but we do have a primitive in-built self-regulatory system for stress release: running, or other vigorous heart–lung activity. When confronted by stressful and fearful situations, primitive man would either attack or run away. In running, he immediately discharged the natural build-up of energy and in so doing his racing heart and laboured breathing eased, and with physiological control came mental and physical equilibrium.

It is not socially acceptable for us to react with frenzied rage or to just get up and spring away from immediate demands and commitments, but we *can* still run or exercise vigorously—if we put aside the time—and work off our anxieties, fears and tensions and feel 'good' again. However, all too often we are prevented from doing this by our negative addictions: tobacco, alcohol and overeating all greatly inhibit our capacity for effective stress release. They may give us momentary feelings of pleasure and an illusion of being in control, but the reality is that they only

The Symptoms and Warning Signs of Stress

- Irritability
- Restlessness and fatigue
- Sleeping badly
- Psychosomatic ailments: palpitations, indigestion, late periods and menstrual problems, headache, muscle pains, constipation/diarrhoea, rashes and 'allergic reactions'
- Compulsive eating and starving
- Increase in drinking alcohol
- Increase in smoking
- Overreaction to relatively trivial situations
- Loss of enjoyment of life
- Feeling permanently tense and worried
- Inability to concentrate on one thing at a time

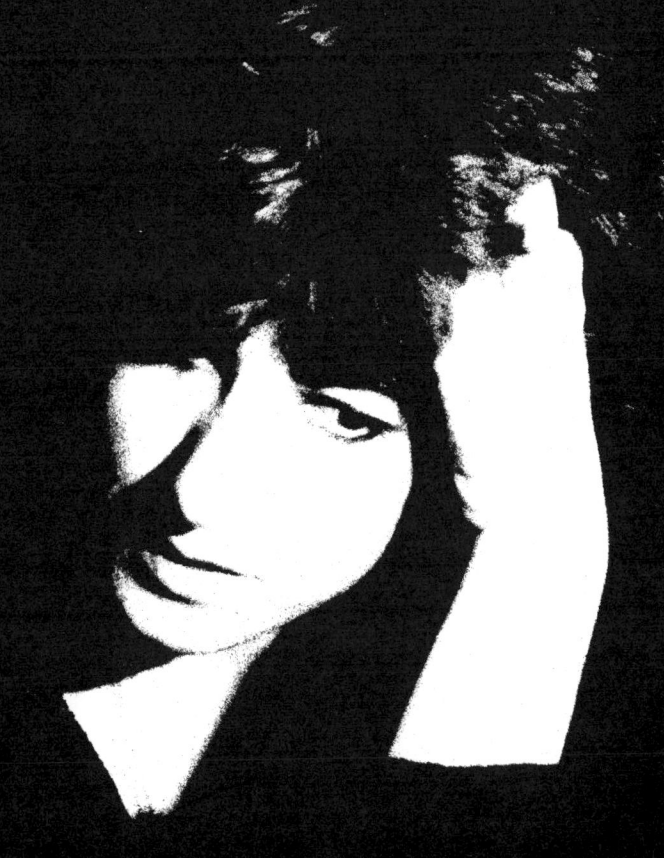

STRESS AND ADDICTION

deaden and depress us, inhibit distraction from unremitting self-analysis and criticism and reinforce our feelings of inadequacy and powerlessness, making us even more vulnerable to stress.

How Exercise Helps Cope with Stress
● Reduces anxiety level by discharging energy in a socially acceptable form
● Builds up physical fitness and stamina
● Allows for the release of tension, offers distraction from problems and so reduces the risk of psychological illness
● Counteracts the metabolic effects of stress
● Encourages re-evaluation of sleeping, eating, drinking and smoking habits
● Necessitates basic discipline which in turn strengthens the ability for achievement and fosters determination to kick negative addictions

Smoking

Far fewer women have been giving up smoking than men despite the fact that it is still the major cause of illness and premature death in the West. Whatever the reasons that keep women smoking, the fact remains that each cigarette you smoke shortens your life by five minutes.

The basic problem is nicotine. Nicotine is powerfully addicting: 6–8 times more so than alcohol, and there can be little doubt that if nicotine wasn't present in tobacco, people wouldn't smoke. But that's not all. When you light a cigarette and inhale the smoke you are exposing your *body* to over 2000 chemical agents—some cancer-initiating (carcinogenic) and some cancer-promoting (co-carcinogens). And these are absorbed not just through your lungs, but also through your skin and glands in your mouth and gut.

What is in Cigarettes?

The three major constituents of burning tobacco are nicotine, tar and carbon monoxide.

Nicotine is essentially a stimulant although it both stimulates and blocks the actions of the autonomic (involuntary) nervous system. It stimulates the release of adrenalin which directly or indirectly has the following effects: alerts the brain, increases cardiac output, raises blood pressure, constricts blood vessels, slows down the rate at which blood gets back to the heart, slows down the rate at which food is emptied from the stomach and wastes are expelled from the bowel, raises the blood level of fatty acids and glucose, and inhibits the production of urine.

Tar, the by-product of burning tobacco, probably causes the most damage because it is such a pernicious irritant. Tar inflames the lining of the lung's bronchioles (air passages) making you more prone to chest infections and eventually creating a raw area vulnerable to the carcinogens in the smoke. Smoking also accelerates the ageing changes in the lungs causing a decrease in the vital capacity—ie, lungfuls of air, and a fall in the amount of oxygen they can hold and effectively utilise. All these factors quickly predispose to chronic lung disease.

Carbon monoxide is a potentially lethal gas that has a great affinity for oxygen. Each time you inhale, you are actively depriving your brain, blood and tissues of oxygen. Since many women have a lower oxygen capacity compared to men anyway—frequently exacerbated by low-grade anaemia—the added implications of the effects of carbon monoxide are obvious.

The Effects of Smoking

The catalogue of smoking-related diseases highlights both the senselessness of the habit and the power of addiction: cancers—of the lung, mouth, lip, pharynx, larynx, pancreas, bladder, cervix, rectum; heart disease; chest diseases—chronic bronchitis, emphysema; stomach and duodenal ulcers; and there is even a link between smoking and death from alcoholic liver cirrhosis.

Smoking Can Cause

- Cancer of the Lung
- Cancer of the Mouth
- Cancer of the Lip
- Cancer of the Pharynx
- Cancer of the Larynx
- Cancer of the Pancreas
- Cancer of the Bladder
- Cancer of the Cervix
- Cancer of the Rectum
- Heart Disease
- Chronic Bronchitis
- Emphysema
- Stomach Ulcers
- Duodenal Ulcers

The Pill: The metabolic effects of smoking are many, but perhaps of most significance to young women is the increase in blood fatty acids—eg, cholesterol. Pre-menopausal women are normally protected from heart disease by their circulating levels of oestrogen (which facilitates the removal of fats from the blood) and substances called high-density lipoproteins (HDL). The oral contraceptive pill markedly alters the level of hormones and other substances in the body such that it makes smoking even more dangerous. Women who smoke *and* take the Pill have 40 times the risk of a heart attack and 22 times the risk of stroke compared with Pill-users who don't smoke. In fact, Dr John Guillebaud, an expert on the Pill, says: 'Ideally, no Pill-user, whether aged 20 or 35, should ever smoke cigarettes.' So, female smokers who are sexually active are, by virtue of their habit, denying themselves the most effective form of contraception. Ironically, perhaps, smoking also accelerates the arrival of the menopause.

Vitamin Deficiency: Another metabolic effect of smoking is that it robs the body of vitamins and, very possibly, other nutrients too. Smokers are particularly prone to vitamin B_{12} C and E deficiency. The effects of this on women's health—anaemia, PMT for example—are only speculative at present, but worthy of investigation.

Miscarriage and Infant Deaths: Women who smoke during pregnancy have at least twice the risk of miscarriage, twice as many low birth-weight babies (leading to significantly more still-births), and one-third greater perinatal mortality rate (death in the first month of life). The effects of smoking on the foetus are as follows:

First, since nicotine is a potent constrictor of blood vessels, it narrows the maternal blood supply to the uterus and placenta and so reduces the amount of blood—and therefore oxygen and nourishment—reaching the baby. Second, nicotine crosses the placental barrier, enters the foetal circulation and—theoretically, at least, but no one knows exactly how—directly affects the foetal organs. Third, carbon monoxide competes with and triumphs over oxygen for a place on the haemoglobin molecule, reducing still further the amount of oxygen the baby receives.

But the effect of smoking on babies doesn't stop with delivery. High concentrations of nicotine are present in the breastmilk of smokers, and in households where the parents smoke, there is an increased risk of pneumonia and bronchitis in young children—particularly in their first year.

Loneliness: Later in life, according to a report from the Yale University School of Nursing, women who smoked were 'more restricted in activity, suffered more from loneliness and depression, and felt ill more often'.

Positive Addiction

Obviously, you can only stop smoking if you want to, and while some treatments work because they offer safer alternatives (eg, nicotine chewing gum), the real answer lies in replacing this negative addiction with a positive one. Many women have successfully quit smoking by taking up jogging or an exercise programme. This allowed them to drain off their frustrations, gave a renewed sense of self-worth and, because they appreciated their fitter bodies, made them realise that they could not—and did not need to—go on abusing themselves. Running, for example, releases pleasure-giving opiate substances in the brain. This gives the runner (and jogger!) a sense of inner peace, satisfaction and even euphoria that far surpasses any artificial buzz or high. Furthermore, the deep, measured breathing involved in running or jogging rapidly cancels the need for cigarettes.

Weight Gain: The risk of gaining weight after stopping smoking needs some explaining. First, nicotine is an appetite suppressant, so once you stop smoking, your appetite returns. Second, whatever the reasons for smoking, one of its obvious pleasures is oral satisfaction. Remove the cigarettes from the mouth and this urge becomes frustrated, but can then be quelled either by eating, drinking or chewing (eg, gum). Third, smoking is a psychological prop. Remove this prop at times of even mild stress, and the smoker panics in a bid to find another crutch. Often, because of taking up an exercise programme, no prop is needed as this person finds new strengths within herself. But if there is no such mechanism then the person may well turn to alcohol or food for support. If food, then weight gain is inevitable, although it is often short term and can be helped by exercise. Think back to your eating habits before you smoked.

Alcohol

Many women use alcohol to try and cope with personal and emotional stresses and strains. It is now socially acceptable for women to drink 'moderately' but the three-fold increase in women's drinking in the past ten years, far from helping with problems, has actually brought problems of its own.

Alcohol in Your Body

Alcohol is quickly absorbed from the stomach and gut and carried in the bloodstream to every part of the body. In the brain, it acts as a depressant, shutting off the higher brain centres and leaving you relaxed and less inhibited. But it also lessens your judgement, manual skills (eg, driving) become clumsier, and you may find yourself saying things that you didn't want to or becoming argumentative with a friend or lover.

Ninety per cent of alcohol is broken down by the liver. The rest is eliminated via the skin, lungs and kidneys. Generally, it takes one hour for your liver to metabolise one unit of alcohol— ie, $\frac{1}{2}$ pint (or can) of beer, a glass of wine, or a shot of spirits—and one hour per unit of alcohol to sober up. The rate at which you absorb, and the ability of your body to handle alcohol depends on several factors: your height and weight, your health and level of fitness, whether or not there is food in your stomach whether you smoke, your general mood, and your sex.

Alcohol and Women's Health

Alcohol has greater deleterious effects on women than on men. Fatty tissue (of which women have more than men) is relatively impermeable to alcohol owing to its poor blood supply, which means that alcohol will remain in the bloodstream longer. Since women have a greater ratio of body fat to water and muscle than men, for each unit of alcohol that a woman and a man drink, the woman will have a higher concentration of alcohol in her circulation. Women are also smaller and lighter (on average) than men and also have a lower metabolic rate, so, the problem of coping with alcohol becomes compounded.

Women drinkers are especially prone to duodenal ulcers and vitamin and mineral deficiency. Researchers say we should limit our intake of alcohol to a maximum of 4 units (80 mg) a day.

STRESS AND ADDICTION

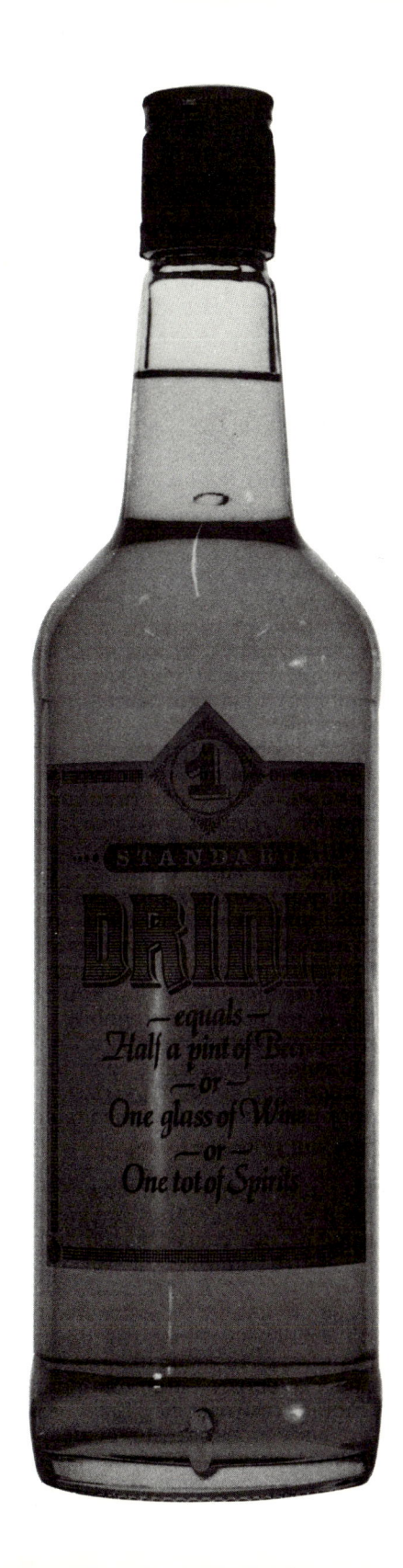

Others are more cautious and say that as little as 40 mg alcohol a day exposes us to the risk of severe liver damage.

Pre-Menstrual Tension: Many women have noticed how their ability to handle alcohol varies with where they are in their menstrual cycle. Typically, it is poorer premenstrually—although this is also when women tend to drink more—and women are more likely to get drunk, upset and depressed, and hungover than they would normally. In addition, alcohol will exacerbate any vitamin or mineral losses, and also deprive you of good quality sleep.

Pregnancy: It is only relatively recently that alcohol was found to cross the placental barrier and—in theory—affect the foetus. Meanwhile, reports are accumulating of a particular syndrome seen in the babies of mothers who drank—sometimes hardly at all—during pregnancy. Foetal Alcohol Syndrome (FAH) is characterised by certain facial features, growth and behavioural problems, and even mental deficiency. It is still not known when in pregnancy or in what quantity alcohol does the damage, but experts in both the UK and US agree that even very moderate drinking is associated with increased risk of miscarriage, and that it is best to avoid alcohol totally in pregnancy. It is perhaps no mere coincidence that many women go off alcohol in pregnancy, and even alcoholics cannot drink as much then as they would normally.

Breaking the Pattern

The reasons given for social drinking—cheering up, getting out of oneself, lack of confidence, frustration, coping with stress, are also the reasons given for 'problem' drinking, and the line between social drinking and potential alcoholism is a fine one. Exercise can do much to relieve women of the constraints that hinder them from realising their full potential. It is also a powerful booster of self-image and confidence, and the most effective way of coping with stress. Although marathon runners extol the virtues of beer, for the average woman, it is merely a source of superfluous calories

109

(alcohol contains as many calories as fat), and creates more problems than it solves. If you feel that you are drinking rather more than you would like to and would benefit from sharing your anxiety with other women, there are organisations that can help you do just that.

Food

Food has always had emotional connotations: it is lavish and plentiful at both weddings and funerals, but scarce and rationed during war. Mealtimes and dinner parties can either be happy, warm occasions or an arena for domestic rows and personal grievances. Similarly, food has often been used as a vehicle for discipline: children may be deprived of food as punishment and rewarded with sweets or puddings. They may be made to eat everything on their plate regardless of whether they like it or not, or hungry or not. For the child to do less than obey, is to incur the wrath of parents and withdrawal of love. It is women who feature mostly in this backdrop and who have always borne the closest relationship to food.

Women are traditionally the providers of love, security and food. We buy food, prepare and cook it, and all food advertising is directed at us. A woman's worth is to no insignificant extent measured by her ability to cook and present food. She is likely to have two jobs and tends to feed her children and partner first and herself second. Meanwhile she is confronted by media images of how she should be, where slimness is equated with sexuality and desirability—which is most readily achieved by dieting and abstention. It is easy enough therefore to see how a woman's relationship with food can become problematic.

Eating Problems

The spectrum of eating problems in women ranges from compulsive eating causing weight gain and obesity on the one hand, to compulsive starvation and anorexia nervosa on the other. In the middle, eating problems may be less obvious (eg, weight is stable and 'normal') although no less distressing. The combined overeating and starving (bingeing/abstaining) feature characteristic of bulimia nervosa is probably a more accurate and realistic picture of the way in which many women are driven to manipulate their eating habits, and so, their weight.

Although eating problems may appear under different guises, they do share a variety of features in common. Notable among these is a feeling of threat and loss of control when confronted by food. When confronted by food, the compulsive eater tends to capitulate, loses control and overeats—knowing full well the self-disgust and guilt that will follow. The anorexic or abstaining bulimic on the other hand, will mobilise her resources for coping and conjure up feelings of extreme revulsion and denial, and so reject the food. She then feels that she has triumphed and is once more in control. The bulimic will demonstrate both these behaviours on different occasions, and episodes of bingeing are usually followed by endeavours to get rid of the food—vomiting, purging with large quantities of laxatives or abusing diuretics.

Whether it is a question of compulsive stuffing, starvation or alternating episodes of both, the real problem lies in a conflict between the needs of self and the demands of reality. Distortions of self-image, low self-esteem and resort to destructive behaviour underlines the many conflicts and frustrations that stress women and cause such unhappiness and ill health. Very often, there is also an urge to change one's life. This can rarely be achieved overnight but, by adopting a plan of programmed exercise such changes might be initiated. Exercise will also of necessity mean setting time aside—away from it all. It will offer relaxation, the release of tension, and allow subconscious feelings to 'float to the surface' and provide insight. It will also require a certain discipline, but the sense of achievement and self-mastery which ensue are positively self-enhancing and a very effective way of getting away from self-destructive thoughts and habits.

Relaxation and Massage

It's ironic that improving standards in modern living are accompanied by increased levels of stress. However many gadgets and conveniences are available to ease the day-to-day routines, people still have personal anxieties — about home and family, friends and lovers, ambition or lack of achievement at work. Nasty shocks and even nice surprises bring stresses and strains of different kinds. What is clear is that some, if not most, of the stress can be countered by using exercise to work off energy and aggression. There is a notable link between physical well-being and mental preparedness and relaxation techniques regenerate the mind as well as the body.

Sleep

The best and most obvious form of relaxation is good quality sleep. Although we spend one-third of our lives in this state, we tend to be far more concerned with the quality of our waking hours than the value and importance of sleep.

It is not known why *exactly* we need to sleep, but the fact that we do becomes all too clear when experiments are carried out on sleep-deprived subjects: incoherence and irrational thought processes supervene quickly, attention cannot be sustained, and eventually there may be visual and auditory hallucinations.

The Quality of Sleep

There are two different kinds of sleep: REM (Rapid Eye Movement), also called 'primitive' or 'paradoxical' sleep, and non-REM, or 'orthodox' sleep. Both are vital for health. It is during the REM sleep that most of the regenerative processes take place in the brain and when dreaming and sexual arousal occur. During an average night's sleep, there are usually four cycles of non-REM and REM sleep, each cycle lasting about 2 hours, and sleep is deepest during the first cycle.

Our sleep requirements decrease as we get older. They are highest just after birth, and drop sharply after about 50–60. Women also appear to need more sleep than men.

Many factors influence our ability to sleep well. Exercise greatly improves the quality of sleep (especially REM) so that we sleep better in fewer hours. Alcohol and sleeping pills, although they may 'knock us out' abolish the all-important REM sleep leaving us feeling groggy and unrested on awakening. Television also interferes with sleep by encroaching insidiously on the night. It is a good idea once in a while to switch the TV off an hour earlier and to go to bed to read instead. Your brain will have far less to cope with and will relax more readily. Listen to your body too. If it says you need more sleep, then ignore the exhortations of friends—and children—and get your head down.

RELAXATION AND MASSAGE

Established Forms of Relaxation

Yoga
Yoga is the most famous and popular way of relaxing. Yoga is commonly divided into two areas—Hatha-yoga which deals with posture and breathing, and Raja-yoga which concentrates on the mind. This is an over-simplification because the two intertwine, but most women use Hatha-yoga to help their bodies relax, which in turn calms the mind. The astonishing positions adopted by experts and Indian sages are *not* the objective in yoga. It is the Westernised version that most find useful and rewarding. In fact, many of the exercises you find in books on keep-fit, pregnancy and childbirth are yoga-based.

Yoga theory should not be learned

RELAXATION AND MASSAGE

The Plough

Lying on floor, palms pressed down, raise legs over body with knees bent. Then swing knees over head and straighten legs, keeping head and neck straight and elbows tucked in. Stretch body towards feet lifting from upper back. Hold for 3 minutes.

Take legs back down to floor or, if this is difficult, on to a chair or a pile of books. Keep back straight, feet together and knees straight. Hold for 5 minutes.

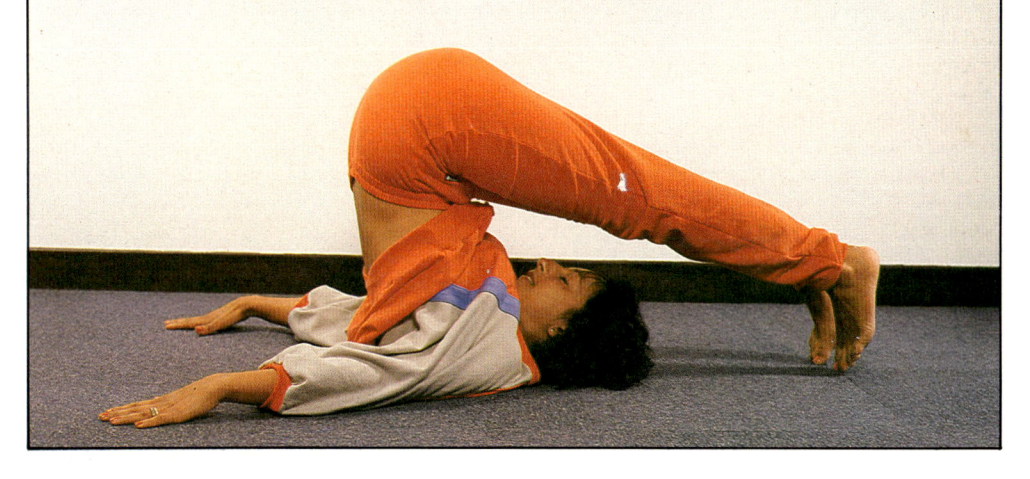

from books, especially by beginners. A qualified teacher who puts you into the correct positions, and gives you the correct series of exercises is essential when you start yoga. A poor base will give you no benefit. What's more, some exercises are unsuitable for women with back problems or high blood pressure, so a teacher is recommended for about a year or so. As with so many techniques, breathing is the basis of relaxation. Yoga emphasises the full use of the lungs which in normal life we fail to exploit. Coupled with this is correct posture and a correct attitude of mind. Yoga routines are a series of exercises, each for a special job—eg, footcare (because unfit feet can create pain and discomfort all the way up the body). Yoga also stresses the importance of the rhythm of breathing which is the basis of many pre-natal classes.

Progressive Muscle Relaxation

This is a simple technique for beginners that is both easy and effective. Some claim that blood pressure can be reduced this way.

Lie down in a quiet room, loosen any constricting clothing, watch straps etc. This system requires concentration and gets you in tune with your body.

Tense each muscle in turn, working your way up your body from toes to head. Take your time and keep your eyes closed. Imagine yourself pointing at the particular muscle group you are tensing. Move up one leg, then the other. Work up the body. Do each arm in turn, finishing with the shoulders and neck.

Then comes the relaxation. Having identified all these muscles, now *relax* them one by one, making sure they are as 'floppy' as possible. Then stay relaxed totally for 10 minutes, thinking of something pleasant and calm, like a favourite view in the country, a field, a beach.

Diaphragmatic Breathing

As we mentioned above, much of yoga revolves around deep breathing to bring in the full use and benefit of your lungs. Try this simple way of relaxing and getting more oxygen (the source of life) into your lungs and bloodstream.

Lie down in a quiet room. Put one hand on your chest, the other on your stomach. Take a slow, deep breath filling the lower part of your lungs as full as you can. Hold on when they are full and count slowly up to five.

Then breathe out slowly, really slowly, getting rid of all the air in your lungs. The idea of using your hands is to ensure that you inflate the lower part of your lungs. The hand on your stomach should go up when you breathe in and go down as you breathe out. The hand on your chest should scarcely move at all.

Do this exercise a dozen times and sense yourself relaxing.

Massage

Massage comes from a Greek word 'to knead' and the techniques used are a combination of the following: *effleurage*—stroking, *petrissage*—kneading, and *tapotement*—striking.

There are two effects of massage: first mechanical, to stretch the tissues, stimulate the circulation of the blood and to disperse fluid; second sensory effects, to alter the blood flow and reduce muscle tone. Massage is particularly useful for women who exercise because it can be used to loosen you up *before* an event and it also helps you recover *afterwards* to prevent stiffness and aid recovery. Sports injuries, such as muscle strains, also benefit, especially when scar tissue has developed or when you suffer from cramp. On the other hand, massage is a specific treatment and so the right treatment for the right problem is essential. The wrong massage on a large bruise or where there is local infection can do more harm than good. Always massage *towards* the heart.

Swedish Massage

This was invented by a Swede, Peter Ling, and involves quite a physical pummelling with strong hand movements that reach down deep into the tissues.

Self-massage

Simple relaxation can be achieved either by massaging yourself or getting a friend to help. First of all, some oil or talcum powder will help to ease any friction and let your hands slide across your skin. Any of the oils commonly used in cooking such as olive or sunflower will do. A massage is particularly effective after a bath, when your skin is warm and relaxed.

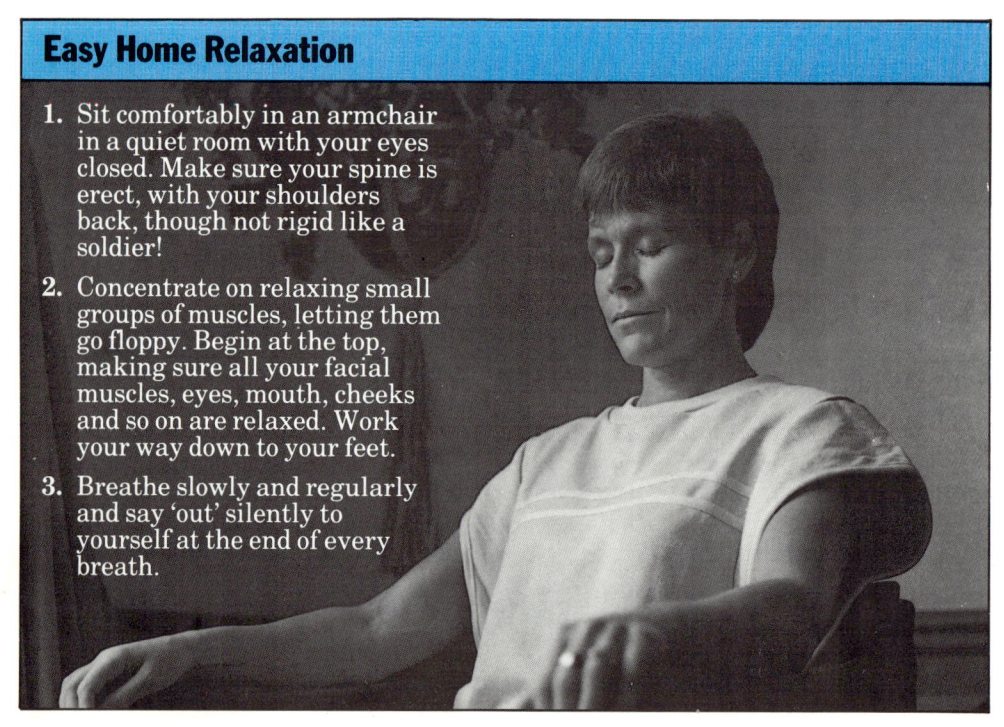

Easy Home Relaxation

1. Sit comfortably in an armchair in a quiet room with your eyes closed. Make sure your spine is erect, with your shoulders back, though not rigid like a soldier!

2. Concentrate on relaxing small groups of muscles, letting them go floppy. Begin at the top, making sure all your facial muscles, eyes, mouth, cheeks and so on are relaxed. Work your way down to your feet.

3. Breathe slowly and regularly and say 'out' silently to yourself at the end of every breath.

RELAXATION AND MASSAGE

Strip off and lie down on a towel. Keep the naked parts of your body that you are not massaging warm by draping another towel across them.

1. Get into a rhythm, breathing regularly and deeply.
2. Work on your arms and shoulders, treating the relaxed bunch of muscles like a lump of dough, kneading them gently. The muscles at the back of the neck, between the shoulder blades benefit tremendously as they are so near the base of the skull and full of nerves that stiffen under stress. This is where a friend can be helpful, as self massage can be awkward here!
3. Knead each foot gently.
4. Move on to your legs and again use the techniques you use for kneading dough (knuckles and thumbs pressing in, using circular movements). Work up from the calf muscles to hips and thighs where the stroking movement should be used again.
5. Lying on your back, use the flat of your palm to stroke upwards from your groin, across your stomach and up to your breasts. Start gently and after a while, press harder.
6. Lie back and relax for ten minutes to take advantage of the effect.

Reflexology
Some experts believe that the sole of the foot is a mirror of the body, and that certain reflex points 'represent', say, the heart, or lungs or kidneys. By pressing the right spot, these can be stimulated to function better. At the same time, a gentle massage of the foot has an overall effect in relaxing the whole of the body. Oil or talcum powder makes this a pleasant way of spending half an hour and should also take your mind off the day's problems.

Acupuncture
Acupuncture is the ancient Chinese art of treatment using needles placed in specific points on the body to cure all manner of problems. Slightly less intimidating is acupressure, where the same points on the body are pressed by the fingers. The body responds naturally, using its own powers of recuperation. There are several variations of this method, such as the Japanese Shiatsu (which means 'finger pressure').

Bio Feedback
This is a relatively new technique using modern machinery, which measures, say, skin resistance or pulse, bodily functions that we do not consciously control. As the machine blips out your pulse rate or registers your skin resistance (it can be auditory or visual) you concentrate on trying to slow down the signal to lower the rate. The advantage is that you can tell how well you are doing and eventually can dispense with the machine altogether and relax yourself when you want to.

Meditation
While most of the relaxation techniques we have listed are physical, some women find some form of mental relaxation most effective. These tend to be based on Eastern (Oriental) systems. These in turn use an object or a single word as a focus of attention. This eliminates all other worries and problems and quells the surge of physical activity associated with your problems.

Like yoga (which is part mental as well as part physical) a good teacher is vital for any beginner as the concept of the various techniques is quite difficult to grasp.

Other Techniques
There are many techniques which involve both mental and physical self-control. The Alexander Technique stresses the position of the head, thus correcting posture; the Mensendieck Method emphasises posture and correct movement while Biodynamics uses special massage and movement techniques to deal with body tension and restrictions. The Feldenkrais Method concentrates on the body's neuro-muscular patterns, with gentle exercises also benefiting both body and mind. There are other schools of thought that involve the mind but deal more with emotional needs and personal growth.

Body Care

If you are exercising indoors and out, your skin, hair and features need extra attention as well as your muscles and physical mobility. Top-to-toe tips provide guidance on special care and protection for all parts of the body and a range of exercises to keep flesh firm and supple.

Skin

Your skin is a mirror: it reflects to the outside world what's going on inside you. Nevertheless it needs just as much looking after as the rest of your body. This means good nutrition and plenty of fluids. Drink 8 glasses of water a day, and avoid too much alcohol which is very dehydrating. Good cleansing and moisturising is also important as skin has a natural balance of oils which can easily be upset. The pH (acid/alkaline balance) of skin is 5·5–6·5, about neutral, while the pH of soap is 8·0–12·0, very alkaline and harsh. Contrary to popular belief, you should *not* clean your face with soap.

Your skin is replaced continually. The rate of turnover is greater in some parts of the body (eg, soles of feet) than others (eg, earlobes). Most of this skin cell replacement occurs at night during sleep—which is one reason why you always look good after a good night's rest. Your skin also has a very good blood supply and so benefits greatly from exercise (and gentle massage) which increases the blood supply to bring nutrients and do repair work while also removing waste products.

Moisture

Although it is 'waterproof' your skin consists of a lot of water and oils, and can become dehydrated very quickly. Even water can be dehydrating if applied too often (more than once in 24 hours) or abrasively. For some people, two showers a day are the norm. This can lead to dry skin unless copious moisturisers are used afterwards. However, dry skin is exacerbated by soap and—particularly if you shower twice a day—soaping is really only important in areas with the most sweat glands (armpits, groin, feet). A warm bath using bath oil is more moisturising than a steamy hot bath with soap bubbles which tends to open up the pores and release the skin's natural oils.

Sunlight

The skin makes vitamin D when exposed to sunlight. If you exercise out-of-doors (even on overcast days) and are not smothered head to toe in clothes you

Sun Protection Factors

substance to block the rays. Most people want a decent suntan, of course, but most of us ignore the long-term effects of constant exposure to the sun which ages the skin, making it sag and wrinkle. Both sunscreens and sunblocks contain a natural substance called PABA for short. Manufacturers use a rating system—from 2–15 known as the sun protection factor or SPF—to indicate the degree of protection their product offers against burning. Thus, a product with an SPF of 8 enables you to stay in the sun for 8 times longer than you could without a sunscreen. The American Skin Cancer Foundation recommends that women of North European extraction always use SPF 15 sunscreen at *all* times, and that black women use SPF 2 to 4. But no preparation exists which specifically blocks the range of sunlight responsible for some photo-sensitive reactions.

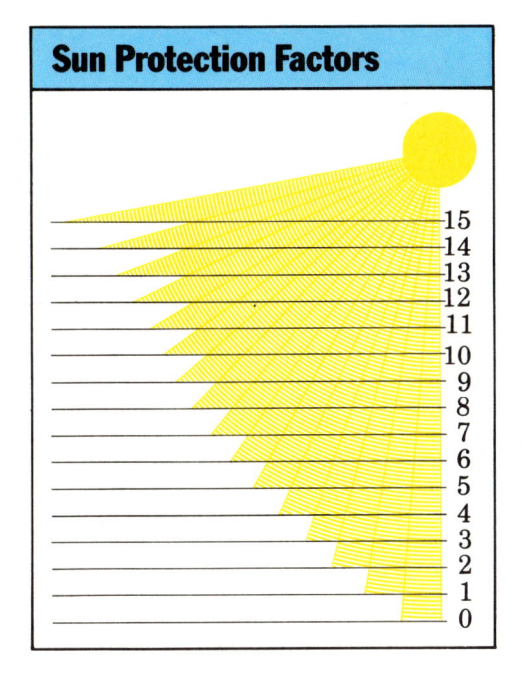

are benefiting from regular, natural and *safe* doses of this vitamin. (There is, therefore, no need to take supplements.) People (especially children) with dark skin for adaptation to sun-drenched climes would benefit from exposing their skin to the sunlight more often if they find themselves in North America or Northern Europe for any length of time. Remember, a wet or oily skin lets the sun permeate more easily. Even the wet T-shirt, so popular as a 'protection' on Caribbean beaches, lets the sun's rays through.

The effect of the sun builds up over a period of time, although sudden exposure on a hot day will cause excruciating burns in a surprisingly short time. In Northern Europe itself the native pale skins have few problems, but once North Europeans go to live in hot, dry climates (like the Middle East or the sunbelt of the USA) they should take special care, especially when out playing sport.

In the main, oils, gels, lotions and creams have no value, however attractive their labelling. The ultraviolet rays of the sun that penetrate the top layers of the skin can only be halted by a sunscreen, made of chemicals that absorb the UV rays or by a sunblock that is made of some opaque

The particularly tender areas like nose, ears and nipples can be treated with sunblocks (or sunshades as they're also known) especially for skiers, sailors and recreation pedalo users, where snow and water intensify the glare. Their disadvantage is the 'white daub of paint' look, but at least there is none of the pain of a burnt spot. Protection should be applied at least an hour before going out into the sun, to allow penetration. Creams have two advantages over alcohol-based applications: you can see where you've applied creams, and they don't dry the skin. You can then apply make-up on top if you want to. Remember to reapply the creams if they are washed off during the day.

After you work out, remember to rub in a moisturiser. Again, this need not be expensive, which is encouraging because everything from jogging to plane travel dries the skin. Black women tend to suffer dry, flaky skin in dry, cold weather but moisturising again solves the problem. If the skin itches, try a cream with aloe vera, the new natural substance that seems to have considerable healing effect. Untreated cracked skin can lead to infection and impetigo.

Research shows that smoking makes the skin wrinkle because it reduces the levels of vitamin C, which in turn takes the life out of the skin. What's more, stress (page 104) is seen to be an enemy of the skin too, producing a type of adult acne that is unsightly. Other enemies include crash diets, excess salt and alcohol. So, the healthier you are, the better you'll look!

Head

Always wear a helmet or appropriate headgear in sports that recommend it (riding, cycling etc). You lose most body heat through your head, so a woolly hat (or hooded sweat shirt) is essential on a cold day. You can use the hat as a temperature control, taking it off or putting it on when you feel too hot or too cold. This is much easier than removing layers of clothing.

Hair

Women who take exercise daily worry that daily (or even twice daily) showering could affect their hair. As long as proper care is taken, there should be no problem. Expensive shampoos with exaggerated claims are no more effective than a good 'baby shampoo' which will also have a more neutral pH. It is only necessary to wash once (twice sells more shampoo!) as long as you distribute it properly over your head. Hair is rarely 'dirty' and even if it feels it, it is only the oil—natural sebum—doing its job.

After washing, rinse properly and don't dry too enthusiastically—this tears at the hair and knots it too. If you blow dry, don't point the drier too close to the scalp where it can slightly scorch the skin. Once in a while, let your hair dry naturally. Ignore granny's exhortation to brush your hair 100 times, it does more harm than good. And avoid using stiff brushes with sharp bristles and combs with narrow teeth. This can scratch your scalp and split hairs. It is also detrimental to pull your wet hair back hard and put it into say, a ponytail because this pulls on the roots. In very cold, dry, windy or hot conditions it's a good idea to wear a cap or hat to protect your hair.

Face

Don't be afraid to use make-up when you go out to exercise if you want to and it makes you feel good, but with the 'natural' glow that exercise induces, only a little cover-up is needed. Before exercising in very cold or windy weather, apply a rich moisturiser to prevent windburn and cracked blood vessels of the cheeks and nose.

After your workout, be sure to cleanse your face (and neck!) properly. Use a gentle foaming agent (without soap) or 'milk'. Apply this with your fingertips and then blot off. (Don't be tempted to leave a cleanser on your face, no matter

Hair Tips for the Active Woman

- Greasy hair should always be washed in warm water and *not* cold or hot water. The scalp should not be rubbed or massaged vigorously as this will stimulate the sebaceous glands, thus making the hair greasy. If the hair is washed every day, shampoo once only

- After shampooing, a cream rinse will control static electricity

- Frizzy or curly hair should be wet with a fine water spray daily to add more bounce. A large-toothed comb should always be used

- Never brush a perm which has been left to dry naturally

- Curly hair should always be left to dry naturally

- Always apply gel to the roots and dry hair upside down to give maximum volume

- Prevention is better than cure, so therefore, even if the hair is in good condition it is important to use good quality shampoo and conditioner

- The shorter fine or thinning hair is, the thicker it will look

BODY CARE

Contact Lenses in Sport

SPORT	SOFT and EXTENDED WEAR LENSES	HARD and GAS-PERMEABLE LENSES
RACKET SPORTS	Wear goggles and keep wetting solution at courtside if playing in hot, dry conditions. Dirt and dust particles are rarely trapped and lenses rarely come out.	Wear goggles because pain is greater if eye hit. Dirt and dust particles do get caught under lens, while quick movements may dislodge lens.
SWIMMING	Wear goggles, as chlorine is absorbed which irritates the eyes. Lens more likely to come out without goggles.	Wear goggles to ensure lens does not dislodge. Hard lenses do not absorb chlorine.
RUNNING	Dirt and dust particles rarely get caught under lens.	Dust and dirt particles often get caught under lens.
CYCLING	Dirt and dust particles rarely get caught under lens.	Dust and dirt particles often get caught under lens as you travel at speed. Sunglasses help deflect flying bits, otherwise tears stimulated by particles can be blinding.
KEEP FIT/DANCE	Very effective, little chance of coming out.	Sudden jumps or moves can dislodge them.

how dry your skin.) Tone with a gentle, herbal or floral distillation (no alcohol!), dry with a tissue and then moisturise with a light, but good quality cream.

Wrinkling and sagging of facial skin can be put off by exercising the muscles of the forehead, round the eyes and mouth. These exercises are particularly valuable as you get older. Try smiling more often too: when you frown you use only 17 muscles, but when you smile you use 43!

Eyebrows

In hot weather, a smear of Vaseline above or on the eyebrows helps divert sweat from running into the eyes.

Eyes

Considering the importance of the eyes, many people still seem loath to protect themselves in dangerous situations.

Dark glasses: Glare on water or snow (snowblindness) can actually cause sunburn of the cornea so photosensitive glasses are a must. Green, brown and grey absorb light effectively and you should not be able to see a person's eyes through the lenses—so choose 'dark' ones. Apparently glasses wearers are not embarrassed by the spectacles themselves but rather the awkward elastic band that keeps them in place. (Manufacturers please note!) Always wear the special goggles provided when you use a sunbed.

Goggles: Games involving a small ball (squash for example) are especially dangerous as the ball can 'fit' into the eye socket, causing a detached retina. Larger balls or rackets are less likely to reach the eye itself because of the forehead and cheekbones. Swimmers who are sensitive to the chlorine in pools sometimes get relief using goggles.

Contact lenses: Contact lenses are popular now, and though eye doctors seem to encourage the use of hard lenses, wearers prefer soft lenses. The advantages and disadvantages are worth weighing up, because while the soft lenses seem more attuned to the

BODY CARE

active woman, they need more maintenance. Although eyedrops are useful, you can use a solution of one teaspoon of salt in a pint of warm water for the same effect.

Avoiding Eye Problems: Eye infections can be picked up at pools and after sweaty sports events if participants swap towels, so keep your towel to yourself. If you exercise in conditions (hot, cold, windy) where you screw up your eyes, try rubbing a little moisturiser around your eyes to avoid dryness and soreness. Moisturiser applied to the corner of the eye will help avoid 'crows feet'. If possible, have your eyes tested when you decide to take up sport after a lapse of some years. That frustrating inability to hit a ball may be due to faulty vision which can easily be corrected. Puzzling headaches may be caused by eyestrain too. Incidentally, most of us are long-sighted which becomes more of a problem once we are 40 or so, but if you are short-sighted this gradually improves as your sight 'lengthens' gradually. As you grow older, exercises to keep your eye muscles in trim can be done at any time, anywhere.

Eye Make-up: Remove *all* eye make-up, properly, every night before going to bed. This will prevent conjunctivitis and blocked tear ducts.

Nose
See SKIN, for protection in hot and cold weather.

Ears
Keep ears covered in cold windy weather—especially when running—to avoid painful earache. In games like rugby and judo where physical contact is made, a headband is useful to pin the ears back, avoiding tearing, wrenching injuries. Hearing protection is vital in shooting and appropriate equipment must be worn *at all times*. Swimming causes problems from time to time but plugs are available for anyone who spends a lot of time in the water. Children who get infections of the middle ear that necessitate the insertion of a special tube or grommet should not swim unless wearing watertight earplugs.

Lips
The skin of the lips is very delicate and they chap easily unless smeared with a lip salve before exercise in extremes of temperature; even better might be a sunscreen or a protective lip gloss with built-in sunblock. As there is no protective melanin or oil, remember to apply several times a day, especially if you are in the water.

Mouth and Teeth
Just as eyes are rarely properly protected, so teeth are hard done by. Lightweight, transparent, almost invisible gumshields or toothguards are now available from dentists. Cheap and effective, they can be worn in any contact sport like field hockey where accidental blows from arms and sticks can chip or dislodge teeth. These guards also disseminate the effect of a blow to the mouth, and give added confidence. The popular image of the gum-chewing sportswoman is also misleading and not recommended because in an accident the gum can lodge in the throat and choke you.

Don't skimp on dental care. Poor teeth, badly fitting dentures and oral soreness can all make you feel uncomfortable socially. It is just as important to feel at your best when you work out as at other times. Clinical tests on popular mouthwashes find that most have no effect on bacteria, while those that do give only short-term protection.

Body

Neck
This area, with the shoulders, is a tension spot because of the nerves that it carries to the brain. The weaker the muscles, the more your head hangs and droops, the more the nerves suffer. Make sure you have good posture and do the exercises which relieve tension.

When cleansing, toning and moisturising your face, don't forget to include your neck!

Shoulders
Many exercises and sports demand arm movements, circling the arms or raising

BODY CARE

Face Exercises

The face consists of a network of many tiny muscles. As you get older, these may need to be exercised for cosmetic rather than physiological reasons. Here are some suggestions. Each exercise should be repeated twice; each flexing or tensing held for a count of 2.

- Frown hard, with your eyes shut
- Raise your eyebrows, wide-eyed
- Screw up your eyes hard
- Stare wide-eyed
- Grin or smile in an exaggerated way
- Purse your lips as if you were kissing someone who is not quite near enough
- Wrinkle your nose upwards
- Have a good laugh!

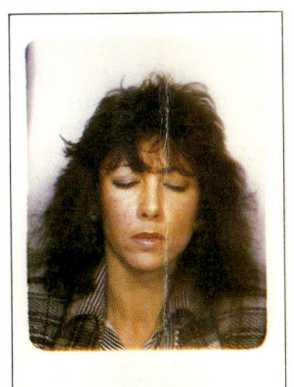

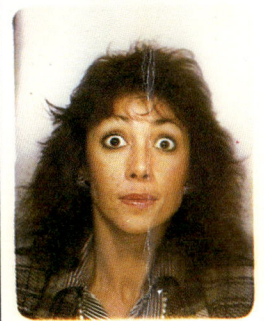

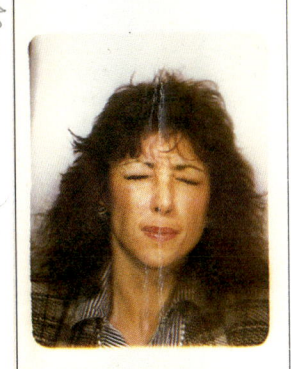

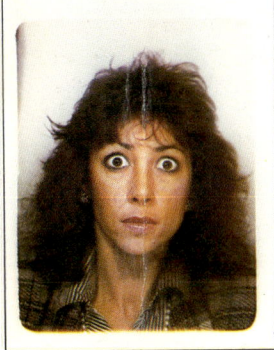

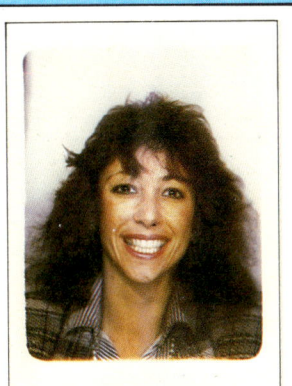

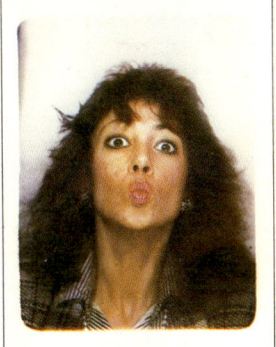

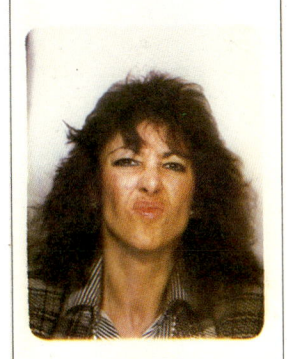

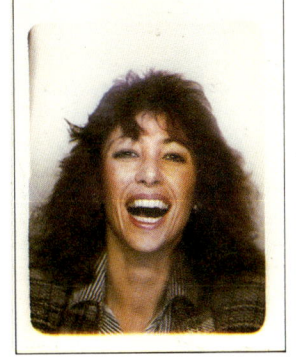

121

BODY CARE

them well above shoulder height. Flexibility as well as strength is needed in this area. Strength exercises are well-known. Events like tennis, badminton, cricket (bowling) and swimming can put stress on the shoulder and arm joints so extra exercises, off court or out of the pool, should be done. See also NECK.

Armpits

There are two types of glands that you use when you sweat: eccrine glands cool your skin temperature down by producing a salty water solution, while apocrine glands are mainly in the armpits and are stimulated when you are nervous, producing a different sort of sweat that smells when it meets

Neck and Shoulder Exercises

Clasp your hands on your forehead, making sure your elbows are kept up. Push *backwards* with your hands, and *forwards* with your head. This gives your neck and shoulder muscles an excellent workout. Keep the pressure up for 10 seconds

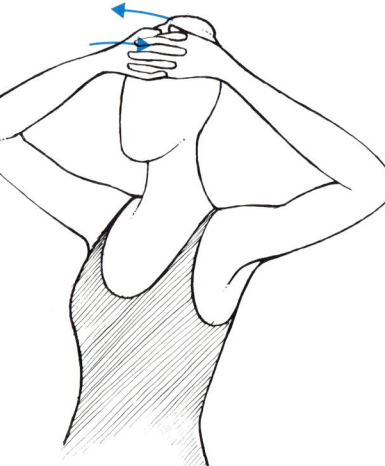

This exercise you can do on the bus, on the subway, or in the office. Put your right hand on your right cheek, fingers pointing upwards. Push *inwards* with your hand, and *outwards* (ie, sideways) with your head. This is great for the neck muscles. Keep the pressure up for 10 seconds. Relax. Repeat 6 times. Change sides, and repeat

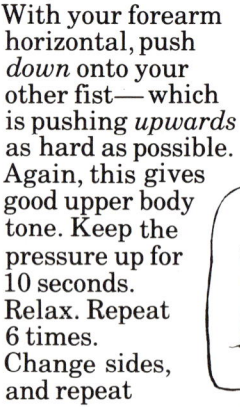

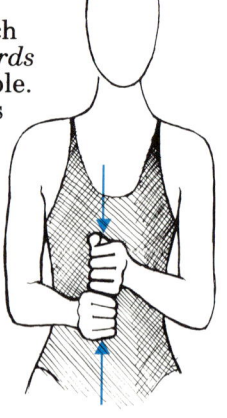

With your forearm horizontal, push *down* onto your other fist—which is pushing *upwards* as hard as possible. Again, this gives good upper body tone. Keep the pressure up for 10 seconds. Relax. Repeat 6 times. Change sides, and repeat

bacteria on the skin. There are two ways of dealing with the latter problem: deodorants (perfumes to disguise the smell) and anti-perspirants (which contain aluminium salts to prevent you sweating). It is unwise to use anti-perspirants when you exercise because there is no reason to stop you sweating when your body needs to. If commercial products seem to do no good or produce soreness, try a dusting of baking soda or a mixture of baking soda and cornstarch. Remember that a dab of Vaseline here can prevent chafing from tight or new tops or vests. You can now buy sleeveless vests which have specially low-cut armholes to avoid that restriction around upper arms.

Arms and Elbows

Most exercises and a lot of sports involve the arms but that doesn't stop one or two odd lumps of fat accumulating. At the top of the arm, when your arms are by your side, you can often see pads of fatty tissue front and back which can be exercised.

Elbows are one of the weak spots of the body that can be helped. The notorious 'tennis elbow' makes two wrong assumptions: one, that it is caused by tennis; two, that something is wrong with your elbow. First of all, tennis elbow can be caused by any sport that involves holding and twisting, so using a screwdriver for do-it-yourself work at home has the same effect! Secondly, it is the muscles of the forearm that are often ill-prepared for the strain of holding and twisting. Strengthen them and many problems will go away. A third factor is poor technique which strains the muscles unnecessarily. More often than not a lesson from a professional (tennis, golf, etc) can correct your technique and eliminate the pain—after proper rest and rehabilitation has taken place.

Wrists

Strength and flexibility are needed in racket sports, ball sports etc, so special exercises can improve performance and cut down on injury.

Hands

It is important to get the right size piece of equipment in racket sports, and the *grip* is as important as the length. Too large or too small a grip can cause tennis elbow. To avoid chapped hands in cold, hot or dry weather use a rich hand cream and wear cotton gloves (especially joggers). Use moisturiser after long sessions in water (swimming, sailing, etc).

Fingers

Strength and flexibility are needed where you are in contact with a ball, racket, club or apparatus. Make sure your nails are cut square and are trimmed short so that you don't 'catch' a nail painfully. To give the illusion of longer nails, use a light colour, skin-toned polish. If the cuticles suffer in cold, hot or dry weather, smear with Vaseline.

When arthritis threatens, put your hands in warm water and wriggle your fingers, shaking hands, unbending fingers and getting things moving again—don't give in!

Breasts

Many women play sport in their regular bras, which not only give the wrong sort of support, but can chafe too. The wide range of sports bras may not look attractive but they do the job, have seams on the outside and give support. Two sets, for different times of the month, are useful too if your breasts tend to swell. They also avoid pressure points (which could rub during exercise) and eliminate annoying and embarrassing 'flopping about'. The ideal material is a cotton and lycra mixture which is sweat-absorbent.

Regular exercise without a bra is thought to lead to sagging in the long run. Breasts are mainly fatty tissue, so are unaffected by exercise. However, the pectoral (chest) muscles that support them can be strengthened and even increased. Breasts should be moisturised after bathing or showering to protect delicate skin.

Back

Bad posture together with being unfit accounts for lots of back problems. Very often exercise can reduce and help eliminate backpain. Certainly, it will help prevent a recurrence. Strong abdominal muscles afford good

BODY CARE

protection against back strain (see p. 82).

The importance of good posture cannot be stressed enough—and this posture is vital whether you are standing, sitting, running or lying in bed. If your head hangs forward, if your body slumps in a chair or in bed, muscles and nerves are strained, causing fatigue and even pain. It is also vital to adopt the correct position when playing sport. Coaching manuals encourage certain shots, moves and techniques to be played in a certain way so that they are effective, and these always demand good posture. Watch the top runners or tennis players, they always have their heads up, shoulders square (*not* pinned back like a guardsman), their spines a vertical continuation of their legs. Why? Because this is the most comfortable and efficient position with the least amount of stress and strain.

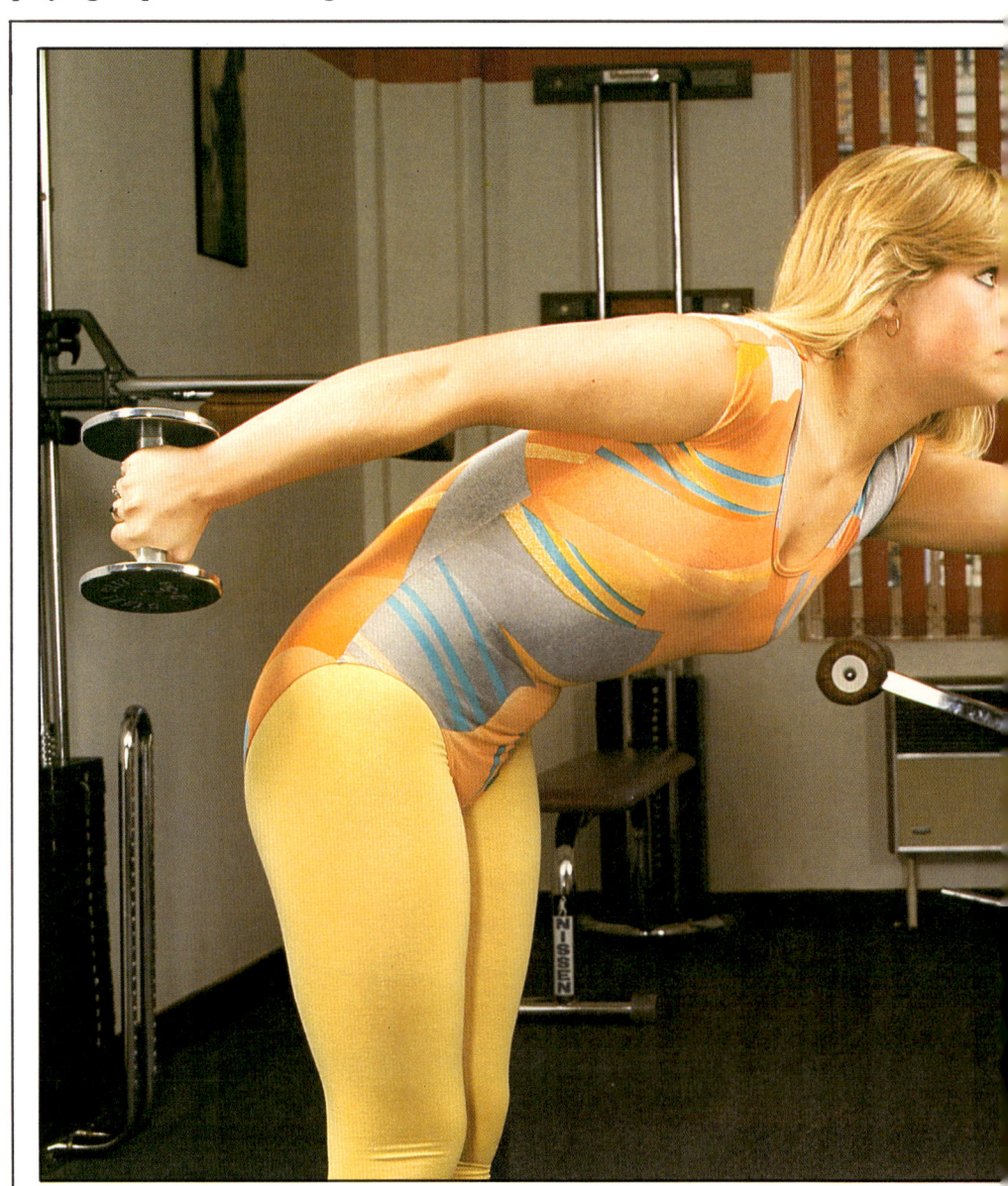

BODY CARE

Side

Athletes at all levels suffer from a mystery affliction called a 'stitch'. Doctors still haven't come up with a satisfactory explanation or cure for this stabbing pain in the side that commonly occurs during running, rowing, etc. The only solution seems to be to slow down (it's about all you can do!) and to breathe deeply to try to relax the muscles which tense up. Also, avoid eating anything for at least 2 hours before exercising.

Stomach

Stomach—or abdominal—muscles tend to be neglected and so create all kinds of problems from backache to constipation. Meanwhile, the spare tyre is everyone's nightmare and yet so many of us look upon this unwanted roll of fat as inevitable. Every and any muscle will respond eventually to proper exercise. Once you have got your posture right (see BACK), then you should get to work on toning and

Exercising with Weights

Weight training offers the ideal way to firm up flabby arms: triceps (left) and biceps (below). Weights should always be used under guidance and proper instruction.

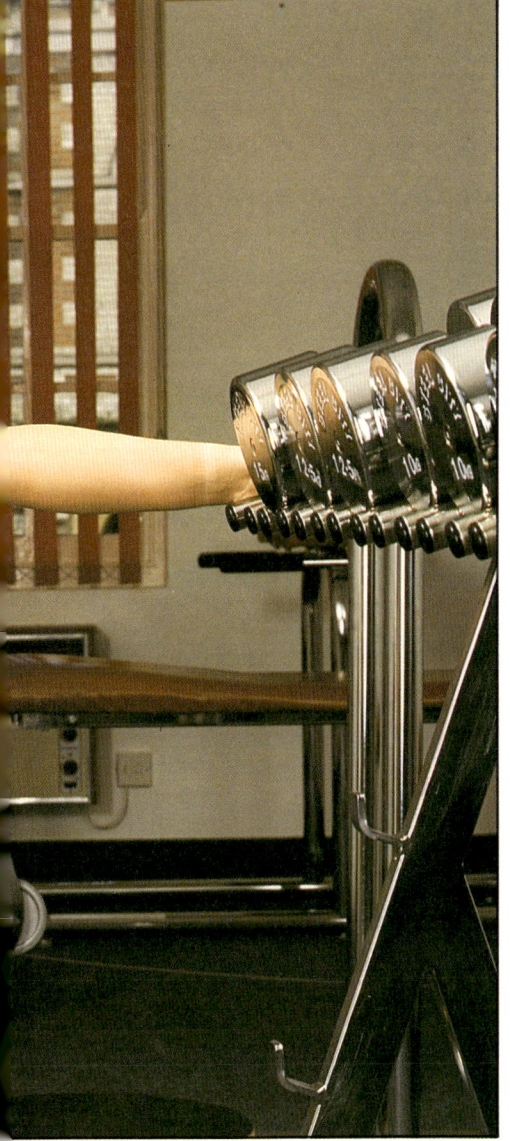

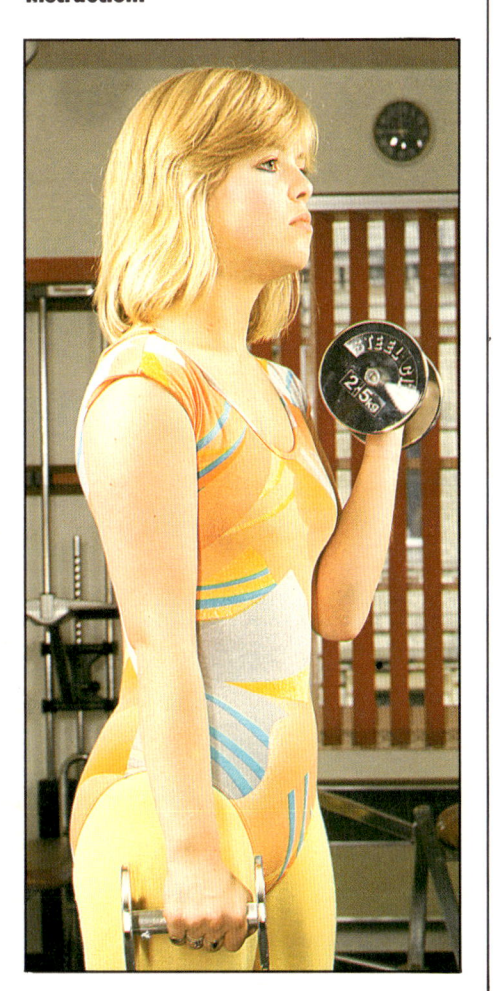

BODY CARE

Firming Breasts and Toning Pectoral Muscles

Also recommended after 3 months following mastectomy

Making sure that both arms are horizontal at shoulder level, push the palms of both hands against each other. Keep the pressure up for 10 seconds. Still with arms horizontal, link the fingers of one hand over the fingers of the other, lock and pull. Keep the tension up for 10 seconds. Relax, and repeat 6 times.

Standing at arms' length and facing a wall, place your hands on the wall and lean forward with your weight. Hold with your arms straight for 10 seconds. Then bend your arms at the elbows and lean closer, pressing against the wall. Hold for 20 seconds. Relax, and repeat 6 times.

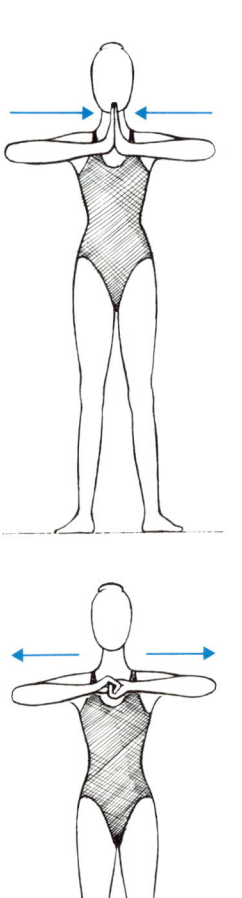

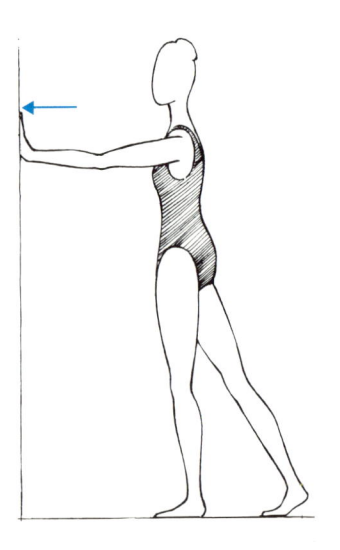

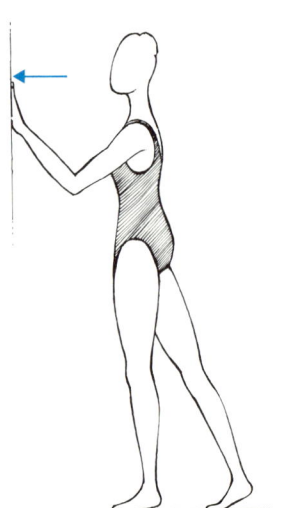

BODY CARE

Stand with your shoulders relaxed and with arms bent so that hands are at waist height. Hold this for 20 seconds. Then open arms out so that forearms are at right-angles to upper arm, and hold for 20 seconds. Keeping shoulders relaxed, stretch both arms out above head in a wide 'V'. Hold for 10 seconds, relax and repeat 4 times.

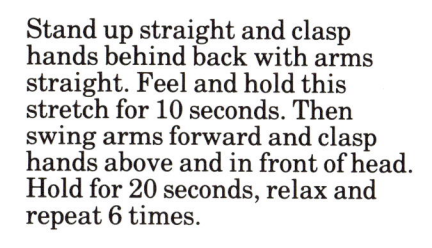

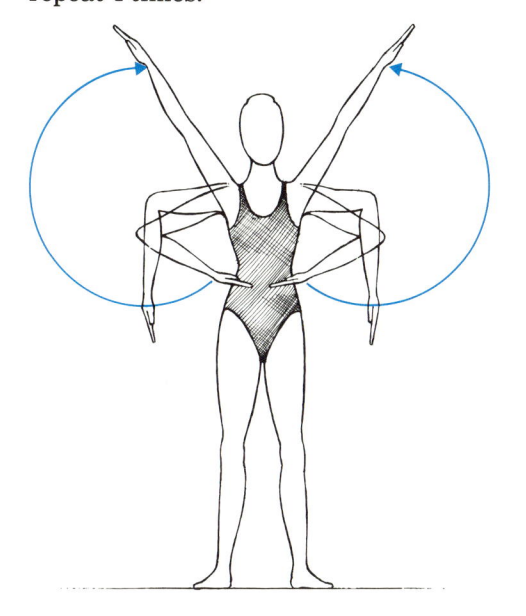

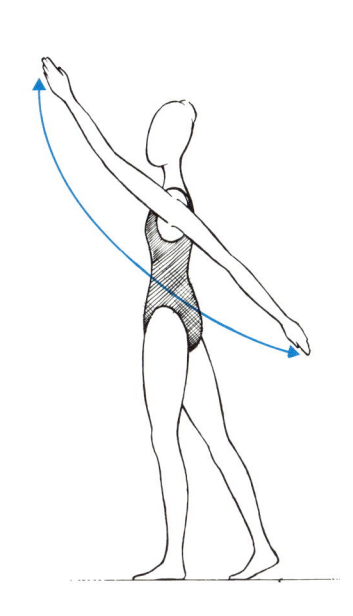

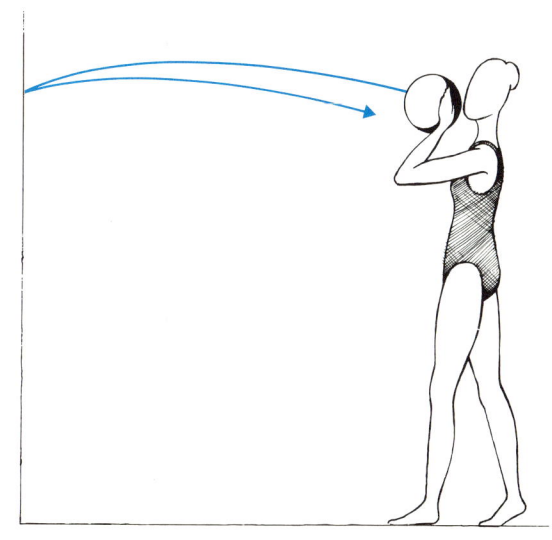

Stand up straight and clasp hands behind back with arms straight. Feel and hold this stretch for 10 seconds. Then swing arms forward and clasp hands above and in front of head. Hold for 20 seconds, relax and repeat 6 times.

Standing about 10 feet from a wall, hold a large ball close to your chest and, with elbows at shoulder level, throw ball against wall. Catch ball and follow through by bringing ball back close to your chest.

127

strengthening the muscles of the abdomen. Remember that diet may reduce the size of these rolls, but it won't flatten your stomach.

Avoid exercising after you've eaten. The body's blood supply automatically makes for the stomach to aid the digestion process, so exercise only gives the body two jobs to do at once. Swimming on a full stomach, especially in cold water, is dangerous. It can induce cramp, leading to panic and possibly drowning.

Groin

The active woman can now get 'jock itch', a famous male complaint. The rash and itching are caused by fungus that thrives in warm, moist and grubby conditions, so always wear clean underwear (cotton) and wash and dry carefully after sport. Special deodorants are not only unnecessary, but can exacerbate the problem. Buy lightweight running shorts with cotton pantie insert attached and wash these after each workout—they dry quickly. For thrush, avoid soap and bubble baths and add vinegar to bath water. For overnight treatment, insert a tampon coated with live natural yoghurt or spoon some yoghurt into a diaphragm before insertion.

Bottom

The bottom consists of several sheets of muscle—notably, the gluteals. These muscles are neglected by our largely sedentary lifestyles and sagging or flabby bottoms are the inevitable result. *All* forms of sport and exercise will help tone and firm these muscles—and your bottom.

Thighs and Hips

Strength in this area is essential for most sports and exercise routines. It's well worth doing special sessions to concentrate on improving flexibility and slimming down the natural fatty deposits that sit on the hips and upper thighs. The inner thigh is not called upon to do much and so these muscles often sag so much that it's impossible to see daylight between them when standing to attention. Give them a workout, because if you take up a sport involving little side steps (squash, basketball, soccer) the unfit muscle on the inner thigh 'pulls' quite quickly. Early on in exercise, before the muscles tighten up, chafing is quite common between thighs, but body lotion liberally applied will solve this problem.

Legs

If you are exercising outdoors do keep a tracksuit or sweatsuit on. Like a car engine, you work better when warm, but if your system is trying to keep your skin warm and keep you going, you are asking it to do too much especially on a cold day. If you wear long socks, take a tip from soccer players who use a ribbon-like tie to hold them up rather than have elasticated tops that can be constricting, causing cramp and exacerbating varicose veins.

Knees

Runner's Knee, a pain behind the kneecap, is more common in women than men. This is mainly due to the slightly different angle of the thigh bone as it comes down from the wider pelvis. The solution is to have good, strong quadriceps—those are the muscles that run down to the knee on top of the thigh. Twisting and turning sports (the racket games, basketball, volleyball, etc) put particular stress on the knees, so build up strength by exercising the thighs.

Ankles

If you haven't done anything active for quite a while, don't be too severe on the lower end of your legs. Brisk walking is an excellent way to tune up your ankles and feet, before running and jumping enthusiastically on them. The Achilles tendon that runs down the back of the heel is particularly vulnerable once the natural flexibility of youth begins to go. Anyone used to wearing high heels will find a shortening of the Achilles tendon quite common, so gentle stretching for a week is advised to avoid injury. To strengthen ankles, try walking with one foot in front of the other on a raised surface—eg, low garden wall.

Feet

You have 21 bones in your feet, all held together by a complex series of muscles.

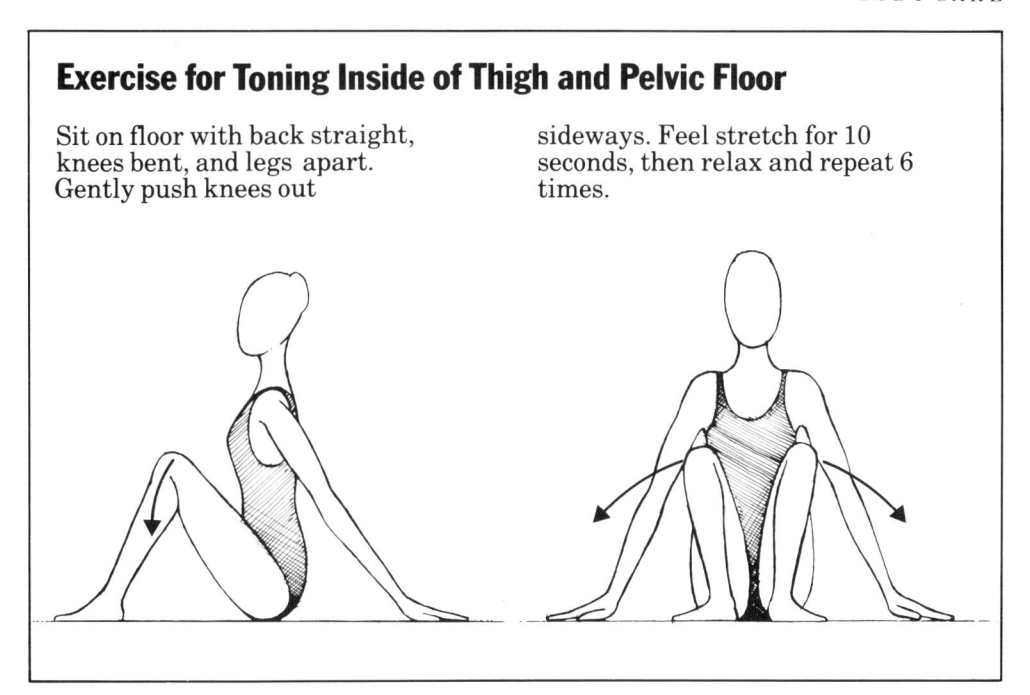

Exercise for Toning Inside of Thigh and Pelvic Floor

Sit on floor with back straight, knees bent, and legs apart. Gently push knees out sideways. Feel stretch for 10 seconds, then relax and repeat 6 times.

The more you exercise them, the stronger they become. Walking around barefoot at home is good, especially if you can spring upstairs and downstairs on your toes. As most sport and exercise is done on your feet, proper footwear is essential (see p. 30). Natural cotton and wool socks absorb sweat easily and allow the skin to 'breathe' naturally. These should never be too tight in case they constrict circulation. Wash your feet carefully after exercise (and bend down *properly* in the shower to give them a good soaping) and dry well, powdering to ensure that no damp corners are left to encourage fungi like athlete's foot or veruccas. If you suffer from sweaty feet, powder shoes and socks before exercise. Use moisturisers after swimming, rubbing them in well to give the added stimulation of a massage.

Barefoot Exercise

A researcher in San Diego reports that keep fit exercisers who go barefoot risk more injury than they realise. As we spend most of our waking hours wearing footwear of some kind, occasional bursts of action without shoes can be quite stressful. Dr Peter R Francis of the US National Injury Prevention Foundation estimates that each foot hits the floor as many as 1000 times in a lively ten-minute workout. At the same time, many floors are not designed for exercise. While a sprung, wooden floor is ideal, many centres get away with carpeting over concrete which can give a false impression of cushioning. It is worth considering wearing dance, aerobics or fitness shoes if this is your regular way of working out, as heavily padded running shoes are designed to do a different job and may not cushion the impact of vertical jumps correctly.

Toes

Toes are often ignored and yet the big toe is the balancing point of the body. Like the fingernails, toenails need proper care to ensure that no sharp edges cause chafing or 'catch' in the shoe. Black toe (where a toenail turns black) is often due to the foot sliding forward and banging against the end of the shoe. Check the fit—especially for running and in games like hockey, soccer or softball, played on artificial surfaces or stop/start games on hard courts (squash, ten-pin bowling).

Exercise after Surgery

Any form of surgery is a shock to your body. The time needed for physical recovery depends largely on the extent of the surgery and your state of health before the operation, but you may also be prey to fatigue and depression. In hospital you will be encouraged to get up and about very soon after your surgery — perhaps even later the same day. This is important because it counters the residual effects of anaesthetic, regenerates important physical functions and reintroduces you to reality. Once you are out of hospital and as soon as you feel well enough, you should be able to start general exercise again. If you were ill before the operation or the surgery was major, you should give yourself plenty of time to rebuild your level of fitness gradually.

Abdominal Operations

Those most commonly performed on women are removal of the appendix (appendicectomy), removal of gall bladder (cholecystectomy), and removal of womb (hysterectomy).

Stitches after any of these operations will be removed after 8 to 12 days, depending upon the surgical technique. This is the minimum length of time for the skin to knit together. However, the muscles which will have been cut through to perform the operation will take longer to heal completely, perhaps 4 to 8 weeks. The scar is made to cause the least damage to the muscles. In general, the larger the scar the longer the tissues take to knit together, therefore, the return to exercise should be more gentle. If you are overweight before the operation, fatty tissue puts additional stress on the scar and you will need to be even more cautious. Ideally you will do better after the operation if you have had good abdominal muscles pre-operatively.

Walking can be commenced immediately post-operatively even though local discomfort will limit the amount that can be undertaken. Vigorous walking—eg, hill walking—should not be undertaken for at least four weeks after the operation.

Following an appendicectomy, which has a smaller scar and less tissue damage, this could be sooner. Gentle swimming is ideal and can be undertaken almost immediately, although strenuous swimming should not be undertaken until the stitches are removed and then gradually increasing the amount as local discomfort around the scar allows. Cycling likewise could also be introduced at a very early stage, again gradually increasing the amount undertaken. Running, racket sports and contact sports should not be undertaken for at least four weeks.

After a hysterectomy there may be some associated depression but this should not prevent exercise from being undertaken, and indeed it may actually be relieved by gentle exercise as you give vent to your feelings.

If taking up exercise for the first time after operation then a more gradual approach must be undertaken. Anything from four to eight weeks is recommended before a programme is commenced, apart from walking.

Hysterectomy

A hysterectomy may be advised for a variety of gynaecological problems and is not just performed for cancer. How you react to this impending operation depends to some extent on your age, the nature of the problem, and the extent of the proposed surgery. If you feel at all unsure about the necessity for a hysterectomy, do not hesitate to seek a second opinion.

There are three types of operation:
Pan-hysterectomy: Removal of the uterus, cervix, ovaries, Fallopian tubes
Total hysterectomy: Removal of the uterus and cervix
Sub-total hysterectomy: Removal of the uterus only.

Exercise after Hysterectomy

Of particular importance are pelvic floor exercises (see p. 80). Do these at least once a day and whenever you are on the phone or waiting for a bus or train. No specific exercise should be undertaken until stitches removed (usually around 10 days). No exercises that cause pain should be done.

The only specific exercises for the tummy muscles are back flattening exercises and these should be done with knees bent (crook lying).

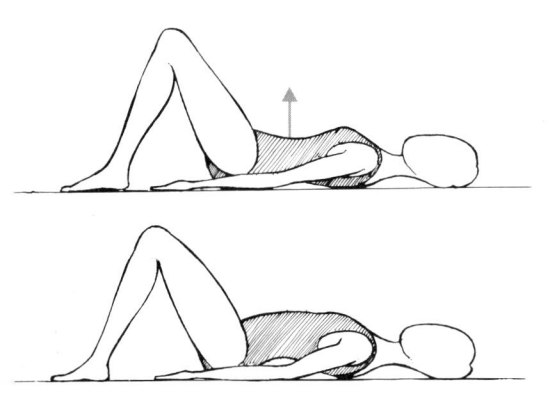

Hold the position for 6 secs and relax for 6 secs; repeat exercise 10 times, rest 1 min, repeat, rest 1 min, repeat.

To do this you should be tightening tummy muscles. The aim is to push the small of the back into the floor. To check that you are doing this, place your hand—or preferably someone else's—in the small of the back, push the small of the back downwards until it is flat on the floor so that it is pressing firmly on the hand. Once you get the feel of this exercise, you can do it when standing (when the knees do not need to be bent). Whenever you have a spare moment— eg, waiting for a bus etc.

After ten weeks, you can do sit-ups. These are more safely done in the crook-lying position and movements should be slow and controlled, not jerky. Start with 5 repeats and build up slowly.

In addition to these exercises which strengthen the tummy muscles, it is important—once the muscle fibres that have been cut for the operation have healed, after 6 weeks—that gentle stretching exercises are done to prevent shrinking of the scar tissue. Initially being absolutely flat on your back— preferably on the floor to avoid sag—is enough. Lie for 10 minutes each day like this and practise relaxation at the same time. After eight weeks you can place a small cushion in the small of the back to increase tummy muscle tone.

It is important to combine the stretching and strengthening exercises and not just do one. But remember, back flattening exercise can start as soon as stitches are removed whereas the stretching exercise should not begin until 6 weeks. After 10 weeks start lying on your tummy and slowly arch your back over a period of 6 seconds. Repeat this ten times. This should not cause pain. If it does, delay exercising for two weeks.

Exercise after Abdominal Surgery

The abdominal stretching and strengthening exercise should be done as above. There is less need for pelvic floor exercise after laparotomy unless surgery has been performed on pelvic structures—bladder, uterus, ovaries, as opposed to abdominal structures.

Tubal ligation (sterilisation): You can get back to activities 10 days post-operatively, or sooner if you feel up to it.

EXERCISE AFTER SURGERY

Exercise After Mastectomy

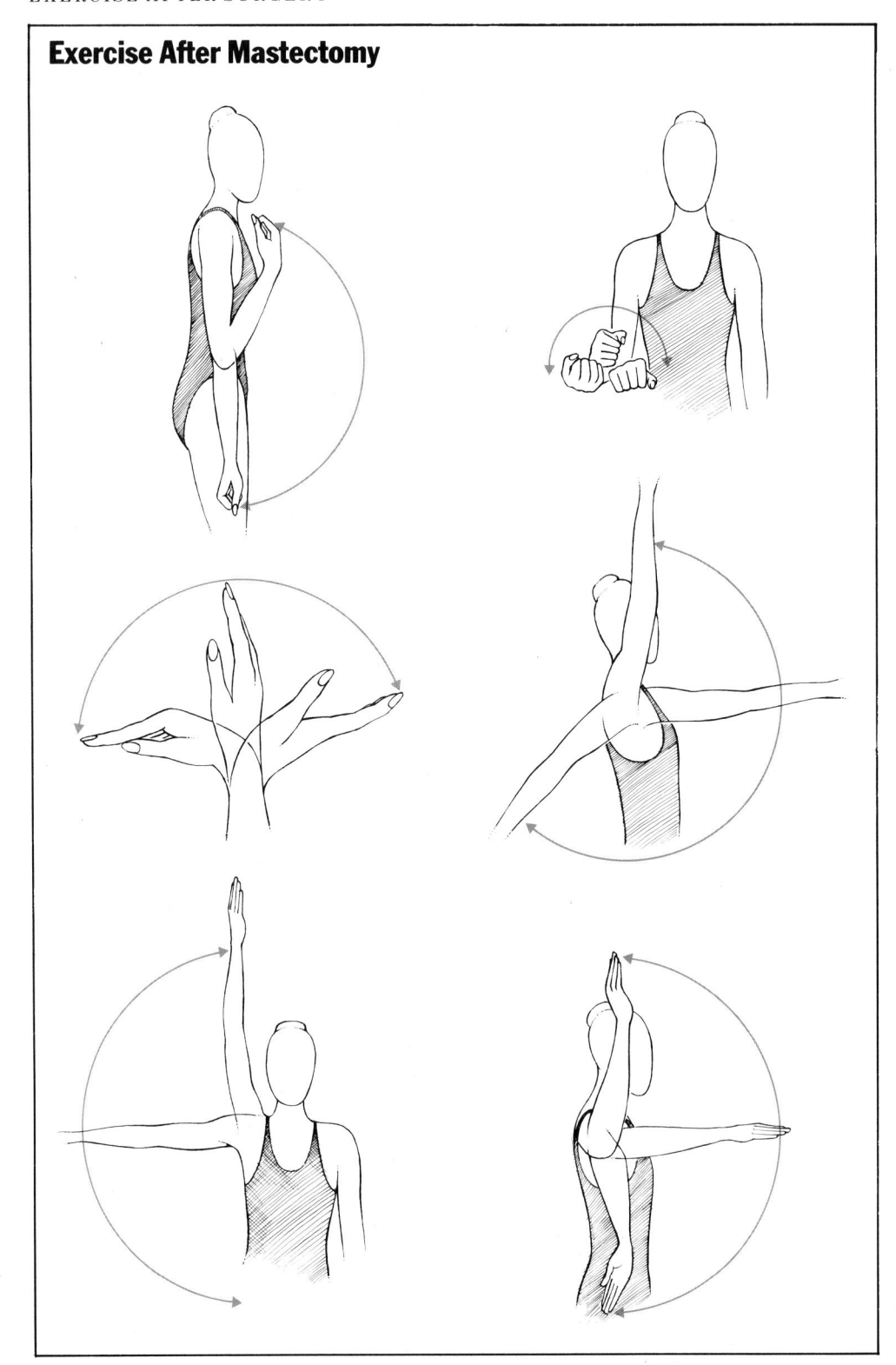

Mastectomy (breast removal)

This operation is a radical treatment for breast cancer and may be combined with radiotherapy and/or a course of drugs. It is a procedure that demands a lot of emotional support and often a considerable period of psychological adjustment.

The nature of the surgery is such that the arm on the side of the body from which the breast was removed will be affected and must therefore be watched closely. Although you will be up and about the day after surgery, great care must be taken to avoid knocks or damage to the arm, hand, or fingers, as this could delay overall healing or cause infection.

However, arm exercises (as shown opposite) are necessary to encourage circulation and fluid drainage and to prevent contracture of the arm muscles which could then limit the range of movement. These may begin on the second or third day (depending on your surgeon) and may be done 2 to 4 times a day. The frequency and vigour of these exercises is gradually increased and toilet preparations, such as hair-brushing, encouraged. Later, a more formal plan of exercise will be devised (such as the breast/chest firming exercises on p. 126) although you should not attempt any lifting until at least 12 weeks post-operatively.

An artificial breast (prosthesis) will be provided to wear in your bra, if you wish.

Lumpectomy (removal of breast lump)

This requires only a small incision, and exercise can be resumed almost immediately.

Caesarian Section

This is the surgical delivery of a baby by either a vertical (paramedian) incision or a low, horizontal cut, known as a Pfannesteil or bikini cut. As the mother's pubic hair is shaved for this incision, once it grows back the scar line is usually hidden.

While lying in bed recovering, gentle flexing of the muscles from toe to head are a good way of beginning to restore your body, particularly if you were ill before the delivery.

Flex your toes, ankles.

Slide your feet up and down, bringing your knees up.

Lift one leg a fraction of an inch off the bed, as long as it doesn't hurt.

Pant, like a dog, to exercise your chest muscles.

Once you have recovered from initial effects of the operation (after about a week in most cases), you can begin gentle post-natal exercises (see p. 84), and pelvic floor exercises (p. 80), but absolutely no straight sit-ups. Cycling is good exercise because there is no pressure on your abdomen, but jogging and swimming (using waterproof dressings) may have to wait 3 or 4 weeks, and at the slightest hint of pain, stop.

Make yourself very comfortable with pillows before you breast-feed so that the baby isn't resting on your tummy.

Varicose Veins

If these need treatment because of pain or ulceration, the veins can either be injected with 'sclerosing' solution which causes the varicosities to harden and disappear (this can be done in Outpatients or the doctor's office), or the veins can be tied and stripped, which requires a general anaesthetic. After either procedure, the legs will have a supportive bandage for 2 weeks.

Exercise after Treatment

Walking is very important, beginning with the day the veins were treated. This is to encourage blood flow through the deep veins of the legs. After the stitches are removed (day 7) you can go swimming; after 2 weeks, you can take up exercise again, and after a month you can run, jog or cycle again.

Sport and Exercise Guide

This comprehensive catalogue offers you a range of different and complementary forms of exercise and sport. Listed alphabetically, each entry incorporates a brief description before outlining its features in terms of cost, convenience, difficulty/skill, sociability, muscles used, wear and tear, and time. Look through this section once you have reached a comfortable level of fitness and find the right sport or exercise for you.

For sport and exercise in pregnancy

Follow the code for the level of exercise you have been accustomed to:
A — Competitive exercise
B — Regular exercise
C — Pre-conception exercise only
D — Little or no exercise
With the letter code is a number indicating that the sport is suitable in the first (1), second (2) or third (3) trimester of pregnancy.

Sports suitable for women aged 50 and over are designated Over 50.

Aikido

Japanese martial art where opponents try to catch each other off balance. Valuable for self defence, self discipline and body awareness.
Cost: Medium price for kit and classes. Important to learn with for recognised teacher.
Convenience: Classes widespread.
Sociability: Good. Increasingly popular with women due to self defence value.
Difficulty/Skill: No specific prerequisites. Any age or fitness level welcome. Develop at your own pace.
Muscles Used: Strength and flexibility in arms and wrists, legs and shoulders. Encourages suppleness, no effect on weight or muscles.
Wear and Tear: Sprains, strains and bruises, especially to wrist, elbow and shoulder. Mainly due to falling badly.
Time: Minimum is one coaching session per week plus own time to practise techniques. Enables basics to be mastered reasonably quickly but more time needed to have noticeable training effect. Two sessions a week encouraged at start, but beginners not rushed.
Specific Tips: At start, do go through with full trial/introductory programme (10 sessions), to put art into perspective. An individual sport so you can go at your own pace. Related to own strength and fitness so no problems for women or fear of being mismatched

Pregnancy: A, B—1 Over 50

Archery

Bows, arrows and targets.
Cost: No outlay initially as clubs give training and lend equipment for free. Often six basic 'trial' lessons given free or at a low cost; thereafter cost reasonable.
Convenience: More clubs than you realise.
Sociability: Very good. New members warmly welcomed and helped by seniors. Tournaments held and other good social occasions.
Difficulty/Skill: No prior fitness, skill or experience required.

Muscles Used: Strength in upper body and arms to draw bow. Flexibility in shoulders, elbows, wrists, upper and lower back, neck.
Wear and Tear: Sore muscles in neck, shoulders and back. Strains to shoulder and upper arm (due to poor technique, new bow or inexperience), but basically, no 'injuries'. Any soreness due to overuse, and poor technique. Nothing lasting.
Time: Basics can be taught and acquired easily but much practice needed for consistent accuracy.
Specific Hints: Chest protectors essential to avoid painful impact of recoiling string on breasts. No sex discrimination at all: due to handicap system and many variations in tension of bow and length/weight of arrow, both sexes compete together.

Pregnancy: A, B, C, D—1   Over 50
    A, B, C—2

Badminton

Racket sport involving hitting feathered shuttlecock back and forth across high net.
Cost: Low. Clothes interchangeable with squash or tennis. Own racket should be bought but lasts a long time. Cost of playing usually low, especially in club.
Convenience: Widely played in Europe and Far East. Many clubs and teams both highly competitive and social. Played in sports halls, church halls, schools. Mixed doubles popular, so convenient fitness system for couples.
Sociability: Excellent. Doubles and mixed doubles are the predominant games at clubs. Established pattern of changing partners and playing all other pairs ensures extensive range of contacts. Players at every level so easy to fit into a club.
Difficulty/Skill: Agility and good reflexes needed to play game well. This develops with practice. Basic technique of striking the shuttlecock over net not hard to learn, though initial persistence needed. Soon able to play in games. Great natural ability not needed, but a fast and physically demanding sport.

SPORT AND EXERCISE GUIDE

Muscles Used: All-round fitness needed. Stress on trunk and abdomen, arms and legs—especially thighs. Flexibility in trunk, back, shoulders and wrists important. Played in short-sharp bursts of anaerobic activity but these go on for a long time so good for heart and lungs and stamina.
Wear and Tear: For average club player who plays 2 or 3 times per week maximum, injuries rare. If playing much more regularly or for prolonged periods, soreness in racket shoulder or lower back possible. High level of tension and fast foot action require fitness and agility even at bottom end of scale. Most common problem—blisters on hands and feet.
Time: Perhaps twice a week to improve as player but other form of aerobic exercise to increase stamina probably necessary too. Two games of badminton per week will not make a great impact on fitness—except to improve flexibility.
Specific Tips: Make sure shoes fit well, especially if played on hard floors. If first club you try not right, try another —usually plenty of choice.

Pregnancy: A, B, C—1, 2   Over 50

Basketball

Five-a-side team game. Objective is to score points by putting ball through opponents' basket.
Cost: Kit not expensive but worthwhile spending money on good shoes.
Convenience: Increasing number of clubs for women players but still not as widespread as men's. Once in club and committed, plenty of coaching provided in Europe. Immensely popular in USA.
Difficulty/Skill: Physically demanding, requiring high level of overall fitness. Great deal of skill needed to be good player. Hard, but possible, to start from scratch as adult, although lots of training and practice required. Requires fierce competitiveness and aggression.
Sociability: Good. Great team/squad/ club camaraderie among amateur players. Many women prefer the closer contact and fiercer aggression

135

compared to netball. Club members always needed.
Muscles Used: All muscles involved in sprinting and turning quickly: hamstrings, thighs, calves and hips. Above all, very demanding on muscles and joints used in jumping and landing (especially quadriceps), also shoulders when passing.
Wear and Tear: Ankles and knees particularly vulnerable to jumping and landing injuries. Fingers vulnerable to catching errors. Speed and constant pressure of game put stress on overall stamina and fitness.
Time: 1 match per week plus skills training session (or equivalent) has good fitness effect helping stamina, strength in legs and speed. Demanding at first, and also later to play at good standard.
Specific Tips: Don't compare yourself to male players. The more physical training you can do in addition to skills training the better and quicker you will compensate for lack of experience.

Pregnancy: A, B—1

Body Building

A muscle building routine that does nothing for heart and lungs, but a lot for confidence.
Cost: Kit cheap. Facilities and coaching now widely available at public centres. Also clubs.
Convenience: Increasing number of facilities and coaches although still a new sport for women. Individuals, therefore, can find most convenient time and place, and work at own pace.
Difficulty/Skill: Important to have basic techniques explained by coach then quite easy to work on from there. No natural ability or aptitude required. Major problem is social attitude: bodybuilding not a 'women's activity'; done by very few women and regarded as oddballs.
Sociability: An individual sport at a competitive level but opportunities available to train with others and gain inspiration and encouragement. Camaraderie of sharing intense effort and relaxation.
Muscles Used: Uses every muscle in the body and burns up fat. Concentrates on muscle development—not on aerobic, stamina-building exercise therefore not for general fitness. Flexibility of shoulders, hips, trunk.
Wear and Tear: Hand blisters. Proper guidance and technique should avoid injuries because most activities and repetitions with submaximal loads. This should not overstress the body.
Time: Enormous, if to be done competitively.
Specific Tips: Very important to have sound coaching from start to avoid injury and potential damage. Because all aspects of training and sport itself are adjustable, account is taken of women's physical potential.

Bowls/Bowling

Bowls on carpet or lawn; tenpin bowling on wooden lane.
Cost—Bowls: Cheap to join club and borrow bowls. **Bowling:** Not expensive. Special shoes and balls can be hired each time.
Convenience—Bowls: Many clubs all over Britain and Commonwealth countries. Now flourishing indoors as well. **Bowling:** Numerous alleys/centres in every major city.
Difficulty/Skill: No prior experience needed. No specific skills needed to start. Basic techniques easy to learn and the more you practice the better you get. In bowls, skill, accuracy and tactics are paramount.
Sociability—Bowls: Rather quiet and sedate. Associated traditionally with elderly but this changing with success of youngsters at top class. Clubs welcoming. **Bowling:** After boom of '60s, millions continued to play in leagues, individual competition at all ages. Very good for meeting people.
Muscles Used: Arm, shoulder and wrist primarily. Legs and back for bending into delivery position.
Wear and Tear: Very little. Regular participation may improve arm, wrist, shoulder flexibility. Excess may produce shoulder or lower back soreness but only mild. No training effect.
Time: No training needed so very much up to you.
Specific Tips: Lighter balls/bowls for

women. Not recommended for women with persistent lower back problems.

Pregnancy: A, B, C, D—1, 2   Over 50

Canoeing and Kayaking

Canoe has single blade paddle; kayak paddle has blade at both ends.
Cost: Clubs cheap to join. Club boats available for beginners to learn. Second-hand boats reasonable.
Convenience: Many recreational facilities available; wherever there is open water!
Difficulty/Skill: Not difficult to learn to canoe or kayak for fun. Much practice—and high stamina—needed for competition.
Sociability: While competitive canoeists tend to be very individualist, canoeing and kayaking is fun at club level, for gentle expeditions and holidays. Good for family recreation.
Muscles Used: Arm, shoulder and upper trunk need strength; shoulder, wrist flexibility. Legs need general strength because they support body. Done correctly uses every muscle in the body.
Wear and Tear: Blisters on hands. Strains in forearms, wrists and shoulders; tennis elbow—especially if technique poor. Overall stiffness if out of practice. Cold water and exposure a hazard if overambitious outings planned.
Time: *Recreation*—should be regular (ie, once per week) for a while to learn techniques then as much or little as you want. Definite training effect of firming muscles and increasing shoulder and wrist flexibility. Stamina can also be improved.
Competition—excellent for muscles and cardio-respiratory system. (2 sessions per week minimum plus strength/stamina training.)
Specific Tips: Water safety vital; life jacket should *always* be worn. Rolling techniques must be learned for kayaking. Always have experienced 'buddy'. Never do, or allow, silly pranks in water.

Pregnancy: A, B, C—1   Over 50

SPORT AND EXERCISE GUIDE

Circuit Training

An intensive fitness system, involving a series of exercises designed to give all-round fitness.
Cost: Access to gym needed. Could be expensive private clubs/hotels or cheaper public leisure centres. Club membership and cost per session varies enormously, often dependent on quality and experience of instructors.
Convenience: Now available in private/public clubs. Provides say, half an hour at a time of intensive training —eg, in lunch hour.
Sociability: Little, as essentially individual. Even if others are around you, you work alone to own circuit/weight/time targets.
Difficulty/Skill: No prior experience/knowledge/skills required. Not difficult to do in terms of techniques; each exercise can be as hard or as easy as you want depending on what you want to get out of it. Expert tuition/supervision vital for effectiveness and to avoid injury.
Muscles Used: Full and proper circuit should use virtually every muscle in body. Will also work on flexibility of joints. Can be adjusted to concentrate on particular weaknesses.
Wear and Tear: If taught how to use equipment and do exercises and select correct weights and resistances, should be no damage to individual muscles. *But* all over stiffness likely first few times.
Time: Not team sport so therefore can be done on your own as and when suits. Can be done quickly with value—ie, 30–40 minute session. Can be complemented by running/cycling for aerobic stamina increase. For marked training effect, greater flexibility, strength and muscle tone, sessions should be twice a week.
Specific Tips: *NB*—Get initial instruction from experienced tutor. Getting correct weights, number of repetitions and positions is very important to avoid injury and achieve objective. Do not be put off by fact that it is still a male dominated area.

Pregnancy: A—1

137

Climbing

Can be recreational or as tough as mountaineering.
Costs: High because equipment of good quality essential. Travel to sites can be high; accommodation required. Expert tuition at length vital.
Convenience: Dependent on where you live as to how far you need to travel. However special artificial practice 'walls' being built now in towns.
Difficulty/Skill: Considerable technique to be learnt before starting but no need for any natural skills/aptitude except perhaps balance, courage and confidence.
Sociability: Numbers small but sense of danger and intense concentration while climbing leads to good relaxation when climbing over.
Muscles Used: All-over strength and flexibility needed—particularly hands, forearms and shoulders. Stamina needed for long sessions.
Wear and Tear: Bruises, bumps, grazes and cuts inevitable. Minor overall tiredness and joint aches common. Most injuries from falls or falling rock, but rare.
Time: Climbing takes a long time, so does learning and improving techniques. Travel to venues may be long as well.
Specific Tips: Technique especially important for women to compensate lack of strength. Any extra strengthening of arms and shoulders very beneficial. However, low centre of gravity and natural balance make women outstanding at this sport.

Cricket

11-a-side bat and ball game involving batting, bowling, catching and throwing.
Cost: Expensive, especially due to travel and equipment, though clubs have own bats, pads, etc.
Convenience: Increasing number of clubs, but more needed and usually have to travel to get there. Women's clubs separate from men's at present.
Difficulty/Skill: Good eye/hand co-ordination needed, and quick reactions, but no particular skills. Clubs very keen for new members. Do not have to be proven sportswoman, even though techniques and rules complex.
Sociability: Very good camaraderie. Good chance to get to top, since a minor sport.
Muscles Used: Vary dependent on job. *Batsman*—forearms, wrists, shoulders, back; *Bowler*—legs, back, shoulders, arms, trunk; *Wicket Keeper*—neck, back and legs (especially quadriceps and hamstrings); *Fielding/running/throwing*—all over fitness; protracted, but low level, stamina.
Wear and Tear: Bowling and fielding injuries due to basic lack of fitness and warm-up (sudden movements with cold muscles). Also overstress by bowling too fast or throwing too hard—arms, shoulder, lower back especially. Injuries due to sudden changes of direction in hamstring/quadriceps/calves. Finger/hand injuries due to being hit by ball. Also bruised forearms, chest, legs, feet.
Time: Large amount needed for practice and playing—even socially. To play better, many hours practice needed in addition to long matches. An 'all-day' sport.
Specific Tips: Fitness usually ignored. Rapid improvement in game and certainly more enjoyable if fitter. Wear and use correct and comfortable equipment.

Pregnancy: A, B, C—1	Over 50
A, B, C, D—2	

Cycling

Recreational or competitive. Excellent exercise.
Cost: No longer a cheap sport to start. Even a sound, reliable basic bike is expensive. Sophisticated racing machines are very expensive indeed. No other specialised equipment is essential at the start. However many clubs will help promising competitor with expensive kit. Club membership not high.
Convenience: Universal, but traffic may be a problem and dangerous. There are cycling clubs where riding is done on indoor or outdoor tracks with

competitions and coaches but that may not be what you want. Women's sport growing.
Difficulty/Skill: Learning to ride requires some guidance at first but once the basic principles are mastered only practice is required to improve. Also need to learn rules of the highway.
Sociability: There are many opportunities to take cycling outings or holidays in groups. Cycling with others can make the activity very pleasurable. Clubs very good indeed. A good sport for any age: often three generations of cyclists in clubs.
Muscles Used: Very good cardiovascular effects—ie, heart conditioner. Good for weight reduction and strengthens thighs, hips and calves. Does little for shoulders, arms, or trunk.
Wear and Tear: Much easier on the foot, knee and hip than the jar of running. Ideal for overweight women and certain running injuries. Incorrect cycling position can put unnecessary strain on back. Incorrect saddle position can lead to soreness. Upper legs suffer most.
Time: 30 minutes non-stop three times per week will help reduce weight, trim lower body, as long as effort put in.
Specific Tips: Can get cold due to windchill factor therefore wrap up warmly and wear hat in winter. Use warmth and saddle soap to soften and shape new leather saddle. Learn to use gears properly. Beware traffic and do not cycle abreast or in groups.

Pregnancy: A, B, C—1   Over 50
             A, B—2

Dance

Many variations: Ballet, modern, folk, tap, jazz—all require different skills. *NB:* Ballet unique, requiring total body fitness and control, discipline and dedication all year, 6 or 7 days per week.
Cost: Variable depending on form of dance, numbers involved, and level/skill of teacher. The better you are, the more you pay, as you will want better teachers. Leotards, tights and dance shoes only extras.
Convenience: Many opportunities available—public/private teaching/coaching clubs/facilities. Many leisure centres, sports clubs etc now offer 'Dancercise' or equivalent several times per week during the day, weekends and evenings to suit women in all situations.
Sociability: 'Dancercise' or equivalent, very social. Individuals working alone but corporate feeling of heading towards better figure/shape; looking and feeling better. Modern/folk/ballroom etc, also very social.
Difficulty/Skill: No pre-requisite experience or skill at all.
Muscles Used: Leg obviously, but also flexibility particularly in trunk and neck.
Wear and Tear: Only injuries from overuse at competitive or professional level. Anything else is misfortune, usually collision or falling over, though 'cheaper' group classes on hard, rather than properly sprung wood floors, can produce stress and strain in legs.
Time: Training effect—dancing continuously at high rate of exertion three times per week. Pleasure—temporary exhilaration but no effect on weight, shape, stamina or fitness. (Ballet six days per week all year at high level.)
Specific Tips: Watch or sit through a class to see if it's for you before joining.

Pregnancy: A, B, C—1, 2   Over 50

Diving

Gymnastic-style dives into pool only for those who want to do it competitively.
Cost: Like swimming, inexpensive. Coaching at club cheap at first.
Convenience: Facilities quite widely available at pools, though good coaches less widely available.
Difficulty/Skill: Requires much practice to become competitive. Requires great flexibility and some courage. *But* can start from scratch and do not even need to swim! Pre-requisite: co-ordination and courage.
Sociability: Individual sport, but if training is part of a club then all advantages of camaraderie. More women than men divers.
Muscles Used: Abdominals, hips,

back, buttocks, thighs all strengthened a little. Great flexibility required (eg, forehead to touch thighs in 'pike'). Stamina and strength need to be built up elsewhere—eg, long distance swimming.
Wear and Tear: Lower back, strained shoulders due to awkward positions and *very* occasional traumatic injury.
Time: Time-consuming as dry-land training important as well as pool practice. Cannot be too repetitive as tiring.
Specific Tips: Diving itself will not substantially improve stamina. If serious, be sure to get good coaching.

Fencing

The art of swordfighting using a foil, a slender, flexible button-tipped blade.
Cost: Low to medium as clubs welcome enthusiasts. Equipment borrowed until your standard improves and you want your own gear.
Convenience: Can only be practised at clubs and during club hours so not very convenient. All fencing is supervised therefore danger of injury reduced to a minimum.
Difficulty/Skill: Good hand/eye co-ordination needed, and quick reflexes and footwork for competition. However *no* pre-requisites to start and gives pleasure from 5 years to 80.
Sociability: Good, as only practised in clubs.
Muscles Used: Lower and upper legs, upper arm. All over flexibility required and stamina in practice. Competition more anaerobic.
Wear and Tear: Bruising caused by off-target hits or weapon bearing hand and shoulder. Back strain, pulled hamstring, 'tennis' elbow. Stiff legs due to maintaining awkward position.
Time: Takes a long time to learn and understand. Extra exercises needed for fitness. Two sessions a week needed for effect.
Specific Tips: Wear chest pads to prevent occasional, but painful blows to breasts.

Pregnancy: A, B—1	Over 50

Golf

Hitting a small ball with a long club/stick from a tee to a hole.
Cost: High. Equipment is dear but lasts a long time. Club membership expensive, though many public courses now available. Cost of playing on good course high. Good coaching quite expensive.
Convenience: Available everywhere to whatever standard you are. But as it's often hard to join a club without a handicap you go onto waiting list.
Sociability: Very high at golf clubs, otherwise just individual sport. Clubs hold regular competitions and social events.
Difficulty/Skill: Considerable, as eye/hand co-ordination to hit ball fundamental. Margin of error colossal therefore lessons needed.
Muscles Used: Strength in wrists, fingers, arms, shoulders, back. Flexibility in back, hips, legs, shoulders and wrists. Stamina for long walk on hot day.
Wear and Tear: Fitness usually ignored which can lead to injuries which are easily avoidable. Golfers elbow (inside version of tennis elbow) due to overuse and or incorrect technique, jarred wrist/shoulder, strains to lower back, ribs, neck and shoulder.
Time: Considerable—2–3 times per week—for any game improvement. Little or no real training effect. General nature of walk in fresh air good but no more.
Specific Tips: To avoid injury take lessons initially to get correct technique.

Pregnancy: A, B, C—1, 2	Over 50

Gymnastics

Floorwork and small items (*not* Olympic/Artistic Gymnastics)
Cost: Medium.
Convenience: Clubs all over the country now. Competitions, coaching, and training schemes. Now found in schools and on curriculum of teacher training colleges.

Difficulty/Skill: All-round suppleness essential and basic fitness needed before start. Balance, co-ordination needed. Age no barrier to recreational activity.
Sociability: Good, groups learn and work together. At recreational level—movement gives pleasure to both performer and spectator.
Muscles Used: All over. Total flexibility and suppleness—especially hips, shoulders, and spine. For competition, great stamina needed also.
Wear and Tear: Ankles—usually due to bad landing, lower back strain due to demand for great suppleness; blisters/calluses. Injuries due to falls or striking apparatus.
Time: Enormous, and total dedication needed for competition. Stamina training: jogging, skipping plus modern dance or ballet. Continuous work on suppleness.
Specific Tips: Do not confuse exercise designed to increase strength with those for suppleness. Do them separately and do not do either until thoroughly warm.
Sports Acrobatics: Pair or group activities. Individual items useful for training but need others and professional coaching or instruction.

Pregnancy: A—1

Handball

7-a-side team game with ball. Object is to score goals in soccer-type net, using hands.
Cost: Very cheap. No special kit but good shoes worth buying. Played in gyms.
Convenience: Increasing. Largest participation sport for women worldwide. Widely played in schools and colleges now. Also 'come and try' courses.
Difficulty/Skill: Good eye/hand co-ordination for catching and throwing needed, but beginners welcome as it is easy to start and enjoy.
Sociability: Good as it has a social tradition. Gets people together—good social contacts. Clubs field men and women teams at senior and junior level.
Muscles Used: Strength and endurance in legs for jumping; also thighs; upper arms and wrists. Great flexibility in legs, arms, wrists, trunk, for jumping, pivoting and diving.
Wear and Tear: Bruising from falls, especially when shooting at goal. In theory a 'no contact' sport but twisted ankle or groin or hamstring injuries due to pivoting and sudden turns. Shoulder strain from throwing, noticeable at start but will wear off. Finger sprain or dislocation due to falls or bad catching. Otherwise, few injuries until top competitive level.
Time: Once a week for recreation; twice a week (training and game) for competition.
Specific Tips: If playing on artificial surface, wear sweatshirt bottoms and long-sleeved shirt to prevent grazes. A newish, dynamic sport.

Pregnancy: A, B, C—1   Over 50

Hockey

11-a-side team game using stick to hit ball into net to score goals.
Cost Not too high. Club membership modest; match fee low.
Kit—Skirt, shirts, socks, boots and stick(s); can be costly at start but should last quite well (except stick).
Convenience: Played outdoors on grass, but growing as indoor sport. Many clubs feature men's and women's sides.
Difficulty/Skill: Basic ability to hit a moving ball required. Stick skills need practice. Coaching courses available. Goalkeepers need quick reactions as well as courage. Hard but possible to start from no experience but need eye/hand co-ordination or ball sport experience.
Sociability: Good social game with considerable camaraderie amongst team. Mixed hockey particularly reputed for sociability. Tours and festivals great good fun.
Muscles Used: Calves, thighs, hamstrings, arms, wrists and shoulders. Strength in lower back improved.
Wear and Tear: Collision injuries. Also blows from ball or sticks—especially on shins, ankles, hands.

Twists of ankles and knees result from quick direction changes. Occasional face injuries, so wear mouth guards. Grazes or burns from falling on artificial surfaces.
Time: Often only one match per week; therefore must also have a skills session and fitness—especially stamina (aerobic)—sessions.
Specific Tips: Women reputedly much tougher than men!

Pregnancy: A, B—1

Ice Hockey

6-a-side skating sport where small hard 'puck' is shot at goal with stick.
Cost: Kit expensive *but* minimum outlay required in first season when all kit can usually be borrowed from clubs while you learn the game.
Convenience: Opportunities limited by demands on ice by artistic skaters as well as men. Low priority for women.
Difficulty/Skill: Two different skills involved: (i) ice skating to a high standard (must be as good on skates as on feet on dry ground); (ii) techniques of fast team game allied to individual stick and puck skills. But non-skaters usually welcome and will be taught skating and skills of game.
Sociability: Excellent. Great rapport between new players and old, as women try to establish this new sport.
Muscles Used: Legs, gluteals, hips, abdomen, arms, shoulders, and back. Strength and resilience needed.
Wear and Tear: Overuse and groin and knee injuries from sudden changes of direction. Lower back always under stress from constant stooping position. Warm-ups important as cold stiffens muscles. Calves and bottom suffer bruising from falls or from collisions with sticks or puck.
Time: Considerable, both to maintain stamina and strength, and to develop skills—both individual and team. But recreationally, women can play as much or little as like—ie, once or twice a week for pleasure and fitness.
Specific Tips: Body vulnerable in falls and bruising contacts so should wear helmets, pads, gloves and breast protector.

Ice Skating

Singles, pairs and ice dancing have special moves that have to be learned.
Cost: Rink entrance not high. Skates expensive but can be hired. Cost escalates with ability. The better you are, the more coaching you need and the more ice time away from recreational skaters.
Convenience: Increasing but only USA and Canada could boast adequate facilities.
Difficulty/Skill: Balance needed, but can be learnt quickly. Easy to learn basics with a little help, but hard to become proficient.
Sociability: Good. Invigorating nature of skating somehow encourages a warm, friendly atmosphere.
Muscles Used: Legs (harder than running), ankles, thighs and buttocks. Abdomen and back muscles strengthened. Good shoulder and neck muscles needed for poise. Flexibility improved like gymnastics or ballet.
Wear and Tear: Ankles as beginner (due sometimes to badly fitting skates/boots). Feet get bruised and 'worn'. Knee and thigh problems common. Abrasions from falls always possible however good you are.
Time: Stamina needed so extra aerobic sessions required. Considerable coaching needed to be competitive. Otherwise two 2-hour sessions per week will help legs, thighs and flexibility.
Specific Tips: If you feel yourself falling do not try to grab a friend or the side of the rink.

Pregnancy: A, B—1   Over 50

Interval Training

System of running training over pre-selected distance with fixed rest periods. Done repetitively.
Cost: Running kit, but dependent on climate and whether indoor or outdoor. Good shoes always important otherwise kit immaterial as long as not restricting and comfortable.
Convenience: Any area of open ground: beach, park, roads, pavements if no open land track.

Difficulty/Skill: Basic element is running, therefore technique easy and natural but hard work required to be of value. Use: (a) for starting from scratch—run/walk intervals—target: increase total work time; (b) when very fit to increase speed and acceleration. Very effective, but very hard work. Most effective training, and quickest evidence of improvement or weight loss.
Sociability: Individual exercise, but can be done in small groups of comparable ability. Can convert to athletic events or orienteering (q.v.).
Muscles Used: Legs only, really. Later, importance of arms and shoulders to lift and open rib cage and provide pumping rhythm. Heart and lungs fitness improved immensely.
Wear and Tear: Blisters—from ill-fitting shoes or socks; Ankle—strain; Shin injury—jarring from roadwork especially.
Time: When starting, not much—ie, 15 minutes twice per week building up to 30 minutes twice or three times per week.
Specific Tips: Follow organised programme of timings and distances week by week. Invest in good footwear.

Jogging/Running

A very in-built natural form of exercise. (See p. 32.)
Cost: Kit—Shorts, T-shirt or vest, top, socks, is minimal. Shoes must be good quality running shoes, not cheap.
Convenience: Anywhere, anytime—day or night.
Difficulty/Skill: Technique very easy and natural. Alternate between walking and jogging at first. Build up distances/mileage gradually.
Sociability: Can run by yourself or with a friend—your preference. Fun runs and races are great fun. Good spirit and camaraderie among runners/joggers.
Muscles Used: Legs only, really. Arms important for style and balance. Excellent heart/lung activity.
Wear and Tear: Blisters, injury to ankle, knee, Achilles tendon and muscles due to improper warming up or poor technique. Land heels first.
Time: When starting, 10 minutes, 5 days a week building up to 30 minutes, 6 days a week.
Specific Tips: Wear proper shoes. Always warm up and warm down properly.

Pregnancy: A, B, C—1, 2   Over 50

Judo

A form of traditional combat sport, wearing traditional clothing, involving holding and throwing opponents.
Cost: Sessions including coaching, reasonable.
Convenience: Clubs, coaches, schools widely available as well as week and weekend schools and courses.
Sociability: Good. Can always change clubs if not fun/happy.
Difficulty/Skill: No previous specific skills required. Always made welcome by clubs. Age no barrier to starting. Competition available at all levels plus individual achievements (belts) to be sought. All work at 'dozo' supervised by coach. A very well organised sport.
Muscles Used: Strength in upper and lower body, and legs. Flexibility in trunk and legs. Overall body tuning-up and stamina development, but often not noticed.
Wear and Tear: Usually bruising due to poor falling technique, also occasional fractures and dislocation—shoulders, elbows, fingers, wrists. Warm-up incorporated in training so minimal injuries below senior competitive level.
Time: Frequently—2 sessions per week—for training effect beyond general suppleness and flexibility improvement.
Specific Tips: Start with good, approved teacher.

Pregnancy: A, B—1   Over 50

Lacrosse

12-a-side team game played with a 'crosse' to hurl ball from player to player, object is to score goals.
Cost: Kit not too expensive; need to buy boots and stick.
Convenience: Minority sport played

mainly by women in Britain and men in North America and Australia.
Difficulty/Skill: Stamina very important. Skills needed: eye/hand co-ordination. Hard for absolute beginner to start, but not encouraged enough in many places yet—no time or opportunities to teach basics.
Sociability: Very good, especially at clubs where mixed lacrosse started.
Muscles Used: Upper leg especially, due to need for endurance and speed. Upper body, general strength needed to withstand checking and improve stick handling. Wrists and forearms to strengthen grip. General flexibility needed.
Wear and Tear: Hamstrings and quadriceps pulled, but stretching can prevent this. Sprained ankles; occasional knock on head when stick 'check' misses stick; knocks on fingers.
Time: Game and skills practice would take up an afternoon and evening each week. Stamina and specific physical strengths need to be generated outside the game.
Specific Tips: Wear goggles and mouth guard.

Pregnancy: A, B—1

Machines

There is now a plethora of special machines designed to help you lose weight or gain strength. Some help, others are useless. Without hard work there are no results, so any 'passive' pad or belt, that claims to make you thinner quite simply cannot!

The most popular fitness aids have been weights, barbells and dumbbells etc. The danger with these is lack of supervision and the lack of knowledge on *how* to lift weights properly as well as what *number* of 'repetitions' (lifts using same weight) are beneficial. Gymnasiums and health clubs specialise in 'multi-gyms', gadgets that offer a variety of exercises for different muscle groups. You sit in set positions with machines like Nautilus, Polaris and Schnell. All do some sort of job, are made of solid steel, and are carefully designed to fit most body shapes and needs. To be effective, excellent, skilled supervision is a must. The cost of joining a gymnasium, especially one with complex equipment is high. There are lots of exercise machines for home use, but beware the cheap, lightweight ones that soon fall apart under strain. The main problem with even the good home machines is the boredom factor. Instead of using a rowing machine, a stationary exercise bicycle, or jogging on an indoor trampoline, try doing the same outdoors. If the weather is poor and you still exercise, the sense of achievement is higher and the fresh air is exhilarating.
Exercise Bicycles: Are good for lower half of body, useful in bad weather, but rather boring to sit on for long. Certainly an occasional alternative to jogging, taking the weight off your feet. Useful for maintaining heart/lung fitness when injured.
Rowing Machines: Are good all-round muscle toners, exercising everything from feet, legs, buttocks and tummy up to the back, shoulders and arms.

Pregnancy: A, B, C—1, 2   Over 50

Marathon Running

The challenge of running 26 miles 385 yards (42.195 km).
Cost: Kit is cheap (shorts and vest)—apart from good running shoes.
Convenience: Can run anywhere: track or roads or fields. Many more marathons now. May have to travel to race start.
Difficulty/Skill: Very difficult as training requires tremendous dedication for 1–2 years before event.
Sociability: Nil. Training long distances can be very lonely. Training together can make you run more slowly or more quickly than natural pace.
Muscles Used: Legs obviously but whole cardio-respiratory system—ie, heart/lung.
Wear and Tear: Feet and legs—eg, blisters, stress fractures. Dehydration must be guarded against. Exhaustion.
Time: Enormous commitment: 1 hour per day, plus long runs at weekends.
Specific Tips: Study good book on subject, build up gently. Rub petroleum jelly on armpits, inside thighs, nipples

to prevent chafing. Powder in shoes and socks to delay blisters. Avoid puddles etc—wet feet blister more easily. Women built for long-distance running having a higher percentage of fat. Ultra-marathon—definitely: women superior to men.

Pregnancy A—1

Martial arts
Karate, Kung Fu, Tae Kan Do

Oriental fighting techniques usually without weapons, using stylised techniques of punching and kicking.
Cost: Generally inexpensive. Clubs and coaching can vary from cheap to over-priced private clubs. Beware rip-off merchants.
Convenience: Many clubs now. Be sure to establish coach's qualifications. To learn basic skills and use as a fitness or training method (ie, no fighting), offers widespread opportunities. Plenty of local competition (combat and kata).
Sociability: Essentially an individual sport but can make it develop socially if you want to.
Difficulty/Skill: No previous skills or strengths or fitness needed. Start at any age. Continue to improve as long as you practise regularly. Speed, reflexes and agility will be developed.
Muscles Used: Training programmes work on flexibility and strength in all parts of the body. Suppleness greatly increased.
Wear and Tear: Virtually no injuries in kata, non-combat 'style'. Below competition level, few injuries because every session stresses warm-up procedures fully. Most injuries caused by incorrect kicking or striking techniques. Some strain of *hamstrings*, groin, back possible. Bruising etc from falling awkwardly and blows landing.
Time: For relaxation and general increased flexibility etc, one formal session per week plus own time for exercises. For competition at least two sessions a week needed.
Specific Tips: Because the martial arts are a boom area and there is little or no proper licensing, anyone can open up a centre. So, check competence of coaches before paying any money. Beware those who want money before letting you get 'feel' of club.

Pregnancy: A, B—1   Over 50

Medau

A combination of music and gentle gymnastics.
Cost: Minimal for classes in public facilities; private classes more, but still not very expensive. Clothing—nothing essential needed though leotard is comfortable. No footwear.
Convenience: Classes in halls and sports centres.
Sociability: Relaxed and relaxing nature of medau together with non-competitiveness and sense of physical well-being, enhances relationships with others in class.
Difficulty/Skill: No basic require-ments. Philosophy—everyone born with free movement, rhythm and balance but this is often lost in adolescence etc. Medau seeks to allow it to re-emerge.
Muscles Used: Entire body. Flexibility, muscle tone and suppleness greatly improved. Will help slimming and firming up of muscles and breathing. (Own yoga style exercises too.)
Wear and Tear: Should be no injury at all. Exercise done to music and geared to have people warm-up. Occasional strains or fall from slippy floor (but very rare). Medau recommended by osteopaths and physiotherapists.
Time: Just one, 2-hour session per week has noticeable effect on general well-being.
Specific Tips: Do not be deterred by embarrassment or feeling gauche: let your body move with the music.

Pregnancy: A, B, C—1   Over 50
A, B, C, D—2

Netball

7-a-side team game, involving passing ball and scoring by putting ball through hoop ring.
Cost: Low, though worth spending money on good footwear.

145

SPORT AND EXERCISE GUIDE

Convenience: Widely played and highly competitive in British Commonwealth countries. Can be played indoors or out, any flat surface. Goals are portable.
Difficulty/Skill: Eye/hand co-ordination needed to facilitate catching. Can start from scratch. Training nights to learn skills in addition to matches.
Sociability: Very good as organised by enthusiastic clubs. Players friendly and welcoming to new people.
Muscles Used: Strength in legs vital, stop/start game; arms for passing; flexibility in hips, shoulders, arms, and wrists.
Wear and Tear: Depends entirely on what level you want to play and how much you want to put in. Can be gentle and easy runabout or highly demanding. Bruises and abrasions usually due to falls. Blisters on feet if poor fitting or poorly padded shoes worn. Finger and wrist sprain, or occasional breaks, due to bad catching and falling. Ankles and knees generally feel strain if frequently play on hard surfaces.
Time: *Basic*—One game plus one practice per week. *To master basics*—two practices per week. *Top level*—more physical training required.
Specific Tips: Get good shoes to reduce foot discomfort.

Pregnancy: A, B—1   Over 50

Orienteering

Involves running round a pre-set course finding your way with map plus compass. The 'thought sport'.
Cost: Can be done locally but more serious competition requires travelling costs to event. Kit—compass, running gear including full leg cover plus preferably special shoes with a grip.
Convenience: Good for whole family and may be done at school.
Difficulty/Skill: Simple 'wayfarers' course for beginners don't require too much map reading skill but as seriousness of competition increases so degree of skill required increases.
Sociability: Fair. Better for training—meet with locals.
Muscles Used: Legs, as for running.

Wear and Tear: Ankles, bruises and abrasions.
Time: Each outing is 30–90 mins (providing you don't get too lost!) (plus travel time). Up to you how much 'practice' you want to put in.
Specific Tips: Good family sport combining physical and mental activity.

Pregnancy: A, B, C—1, 2   Over 50

Fell Running
More vigorous running than orienteering but much less navigation than orienteering (except in mist!).

Pregnancy: A, B—1

Parcours

Fitness trails set up in parks etc, where you run between exercise stations.
Cost: None—except ordinary basic training kit.
Convenience: Not widely available in parks in Britain, USA but popular in Germany, Switzerland etc.
Sociability: Essentially an individual effort—although probably more fun with like-minded friends or members of family. Caters for individuals of differing ability.
Difficulty/Skill: No natural powers or skill required. Set own pace, non-competitive, unsupervised.
Muscles Used: Legs, especially jogging/running between exercise stations; also, whatever you choose to work on. If do all exercises the result is good overall body exercise to improve flexibility, strength in arms, shoulders and abdomen.
Wear and Tear: Abrasions and bruises from falls—minor. No problems as long as do not overdo individual exercises early on.
Time: Two 1-hour sessions a week would be effective, as long as taken seriously.
Specific Tips: Do not try the more strenuous exercises at start. Work up to them.

Pregnancy: A, B—1   Over 50

Riding

Involves a variety of activities on horseback—from trekking to showjumping, trials to dressage.
Cost: Ownership of a horse costly but use of riding school horses medium-priced. Dress and tackle expensive.
Convenience: Many schools available offering lessons and horses to ride.
Difficulty/Skill: No prior skills at all required. No prior fitness. Basics soon learnt. Much time and effort and stamina needed to be competitive.
Sociability: Good and participants share love of horses.
Muscles Used: Strength not vital but flexibility important in wrists and hands, hips, knees and ankles. Stamina helped and required for long rides, hunts and races.
Wear and Tear: Blisters on hands and inside knee. General muscle soreness—especially neck, shoulders, back, legs, and inner thighs. Injuries due to falling range from bruises, bangs and sprains to breaks and concussion.
Time: Considerable if wish to become more than occasional rider. Must be willing to ride almost every day to master tactics but great pleasure and satisfaction comes with mastery of horse.
Specific Tips: Always wear proper equipment including crash hat. No limitations for women—proven equal to men in Olympics and world levels.

Pregnancy: A—1	Over 50

Rollerskating

The organised side of the playground fun.
Cost: Basic, sound skates not too expensive. If you proceed and want to buy high quality skates for specific disciplines these can be expensive. Pads to protect from falls widely available.
Convenience: Plenty of choice for ordinary pastime skating but facilities for artistic or speed skating restricted in many countries. Usually 'pockets' of interest in certain cities.
Difficulty/Skill: To learn to roller skate is not hard. No prior skills needed. Artistic skating requires dance or ballet plus coaching while speed skating requires specific coaching for technique.
Sociability: Both styles tend to be individualistic sports, needing individual drive and coaching.
Muscles Used: Quadriceps, calves, gluteals, back and shoulders. All brought into action and used heavily as workload increases.
Wear and Tear: Sprained ankles, back problems in artistic skating; groin pull (from cold start) in speed skating. Cuts, bruises etc, generally from falls, or collisions in speed skating.
Time: To be competitive, enormous time required for stamina building—cycling particularly helpful—and technique.
Specific Tips: Wear correct protective gear (pads, helmet) at all times.

Pregnancy: A, B—1	Over 50

Rowing

Can be for individual (sculling), or pairs, fours or eights.
Cost: Kit cheap, though cost of boats high, so sport practised through clubs.
Convenience: Rowing clubs on rivers, lakes, etc, so may have to travel long distance to nearest.
Difficulty/Skill: Easily-learnt movements, then practice, increasing strength and rhythm. Good exercise as there is no jarring. A good sport to start with no knowledge or experience as no specific natural abilities required.
Sociability: Sculling is a lonely, individual sport but if you join a crew of 4 or 8 it can be very social, although it requires hard work and commitment to do well. Very satisfying to be part of a co-ordinated good crew.
Muscles Used: Calf, thigh, shoulders, biceps, chest, and abdominals.
Wear and Tear: Sore hands, blisters. Aches and pains due to poor technique.
Time: In addition to the rowing itself, strength and stamina building work needed regularly. 1 mile per day minimum for training effect.
Specific Tips: Do not be put off by thought of endless weight training, development of huge muscles and loss of

SPORT AND EXERCISE GUIDE

femininity. It can be hard work but training is to develop strength, and skills are to convert this (via technique) into power on water.

| Pregnancy: A, B, C—1 A—2 | Over 50 |

Rugby

15-a-side game with oval ball, involving running, passing, tackling, to score 'tries' over opponents' line.
Cost: For individual, biggest cost likely to be travel as clubs are few. Little financial backing so, largely self-financing.
Convenience: Increasing number of women's clubs—predominately at colleges. Well established in Canada, United States and France. Many men's clubs still reluctant to have women's section. Any college clubs will welcome outsiders.
Difficulty/Skill: Ball-handling and kicking skills need developing. Speed and physical resilience needed.
Sociability: Club rugby anywhere in the world has always been a sociable game. True for women also. Travel long distances for matches. Good team spirit with own colleagues and opponents.
Muscles Used: All-over strength is required. Legs for speed and endurance, upper body and arms for tackling.
Wear and Tear: Most injuries are the result of collisions, tackles, and falls. Especially vulnerable are shoulders, collarbones, knees, and ankles.
Time: Strength and overall fitness required in addition to skills training. 1 to 2 sessions per week plus game.
Specific Tips: Major problem for women rugby players is social reaction from male rugby players. Physically, no specific problems; game adjusts itself to women's capabilities. Great for getting rid of inhibitions. Wear mouthguards to prevent chipping of teeth.

Sailing

Dozens of types of boats—from single-handed dinghies to crews of 18 on ocean-going yachts. Each requires a variety of skills.

Cost: Club membership high; boats, even small ones, expensive; extra kit, sails, life jackets, trailer etc, makes it very demanding on the pocket but many clubs have coach or experts who will give lessons.
Convenience: Sea and mainly inland waters. Few places very far from sailing facilities. Otherwise journey plus boat on trailer which makes it expensive on petrol too.
Difficulty/Skill: Basic techniques need to be taught and can be learned fairly easily. Absolutely no prior skill or natural ability required—except swimming!
Sociability: Very good. Camaraderie amongst crews and rivals. Clubs as popular for social life as for sport.
Muscles Used: Long distance or ocean crews require considerable strength in wrists, arms, upper body plus agility and speed. Stamina vital too—especially in chilly conditions.
Wear and Tear: Blistered hands, sunburn, bruises, cuts, abrasions. Bang on the head from the boom! Seasickness. Lower back strain.
Time: Recreational sailing requires little or no fitness preparation. Competitive sailing requires stamina and strength plus speed.
Specific Tips: Keep your head down, harden your hands, dress warmly and have dry clothes to hand.

| Pregnancy: A, B—1 | Over 50 |

Scuba Diving

Underwater diving with breathing apparatus. Recreational.
Cost: High, including transport to location, purchase or hire of gear, boat etc.
Convenience: Inconvenient unless on holiday next to ideal location. Diving off Northern Europe or North America or inland water needs considerable commitment to be called 'pleasure'. However, in warm, clear water of tropics, ideal. *Must have companion all the time* plus initial instruction to pass test.
Difficulty/Skill: Requires good surface swimming capability and confidence in the water, otherwise only additional

148

skill (technique of breathing and moving) can be learned quickly.
Sociability: As you must *never* dive alone, you'll always have a companion and you depend on each other for your life. Simple as that. Clubs are ideal way to learn.
Muscles Used: As swimming, but movement more gentle, speed not important. Heart/lung endurance improves as lungs have to work harder deep down. A week's holiday with two dives a day has considerable training effect.
Wear and Tear: Scrapes and grazes after contact with rocks, coral etc. Need to be treated quickly due to high risk of infection. Also stings and bites. Sudden onset of general fatigue, and 'bends', the infamous effect of returning to the surface too quickly.
Time: Once correct swimming and diving techniques are learnt, it is usually a 'day out' sort of sport.
Specific Tips: Never dive alone. Never dive without proper training.

Skiing (Alpine)

Skiing down mountainside.
Cost: Unless you live in or very close to somewhere to ski, usually expensive. Clothes and equipment are expensive to buy but can always be hired. Hotels and ski passes become dearer as the quality of the resort and the ski slopes increases. Competitive skiing requires considerable resources, as it is a full-time sport.
Convenience: There are plenty of seasonal opportunities available dependent on availability of time and money. Resorts all have ski-schools and beginners' or nursery slopes. During the summer dry ski-slopes are now available to enable you to keep in trim and in practice.
Difficulty/Skill: Skiing is not easy to learn unless you are under 12 (when it is a piece of cake!). It requires stamina, suppleness, good co-ordination and balance. A lot of practice is required to master the basic techniques that are necessary before tackling the main slopes. If planning a skiing holiday abroad, a bit of time and money can be saved by learning the basics on a dry slope at home. Due to different hip structure women turn differently from men and could therefore never compete over the same courses.
Sociability: Skiing has a reputation, justly gained, as a highly social sport. The energy expended combined with the stimulating weather create an air of warm bonhomie in the skiing community.
Muscles Used: Skiing strengthens quadriceps and buttocks particularly, and puts demands on all leg and abdominal muscles. Ankles, knees, trunk, hips, shoulder and arms all work hard in repeated short bursts. Overrated as a fitness activity unless done several times a week.
Wear and Tear: Many injuries to ankles, tendons and muscles occur in the first few moments of the first run of the day and can be attributed to the cold. Foolish or faulty dressing can cause extra problems with the cold, as can the wrong foods at the wrong times. Knee problems most common.
Time: Skiing is probably unique in that many people ski once or twice a year for a limited period and do little about it at other times. There are some activities which will help to maintain ski fitness for the rest of the year—specifically cycling, speed ice skating, boardsailing and water-skiing. There are now many dry ski slopes which can help sustain both fitness and skills.
Specific Tips: For many who ski in a concentrated bout once a year time spent working up to ski-fitness before going will pay great dividends. Concentration on exercises which strengthen and increase flexibility of the hamstrings and the lower back will help compensate for the effects of skiing, also work on quadricep muscles.

Skiing (cross country)

Skiing through the countryside.
Cost: Less than alpine because equipment purchase and hire is less and no payment for tows is required. Any clothing can be adapted, eg, track suit. However, there is still the expense of getting to the snow.
Convenience: Is dependent on distance from snow.

Difficulty/Skill: Very easy to pick up the basics. Very quickly progress from walking on skis to running. The faster and farther you go the more stamina required.
Sociability: As required—can be done alone or in a group.
Muscles Used: All. One of the best fitness activities of all. Far less stressful on the legs than running because you 'glide' along. Excellent heart/lung exercise.
Wear and Tear: Injuries occur as a result of falls but these are much less common and less serious than in alpine skiing.
Time: Usually once a year holiday activity but if you live near winter snow can go as frequently as conditions and inclination dictate.
Specific Tips: General fitness training is useful preparation. Any activity but particularly running, supplemented with arm strengthening exercises are suitable build up. Roller skis are available for the enthusiast to use in summer.

| Pregnancy: A, B, C—1, 2 | Over 50 |

Skipping Rope

The playground game that gets you fit.
Cost: Minimal.
Convenience: Anywhere, anytime.
Difficulty/Skill: Very easy to learn basics and after that you just repeat and keep going!
Sociability: Nil—solo effort.
Muscles Used: Excellent cardio-respiratory effort/effect almost equal to running in terms of stamina building and strength and endurance in leg muscles. Grace and co-ordination is improved too. Some contribution to flexibility of arms and shoulders.
Wear and Tear: Virtually nil. Good shoes and soft surface will avoid effects of jarring.
Time: Nonstop for 15 minutes 3 times per week has aerobic effect. Nonstop for 30 minutes 3 times a week can produce weight loss.
Specific Tips: Get the right sized rope.

| Pregnancy: A, B, C—1 | Over 50 |

Soccer

11-a-side team game, object to kick ball into opponents' net.
Cost: Relatively low. Boots quite dear but should last—worth buying good quality. Team kit provided.
Convenience: Many clubs and women's leagues—both 11-a-side outdoor and 5-a-side indoor; 228 registered clubs in UK (most have 2 teams), leisure centres etc. Many clubs in US. Main problem is attitude—not considered a woman's sport yet, therefore few schoolgirls play seriously. Women's clubs often not treated seriously.
Difficulty/Skill: Stamina needed. Ball skills—control, passing, shooting—needed to play well. *But* can start from no experience (many do) because only a few schools offer chance to girls to play.
Sociability: Very good. Established clubs have full social life—discos, parties etc.
Muscles Used: Legs, hips and lower back when dribbling, kicking, passing; hamstrings—running, kicking and jumping; neck when heading.
Wear and Tear: Bruises from banging, kicks and the ball. Sudden starts and changes of direction can pull hamstrings, knee, groin, hips etc (stretching and warm-up can reduce this).
Time: Three times per week to provide positive stamina building results. More running, intervals and sprints if you want to compete at a higher level.
Specific Tips: No real problems faced by women, except perhaps being used to physical contact, tackling, bruising.

| Pregnancy: A, B—1 |

Softball and Baseball

Bat and ball games involving throwing, pitching and hitting.
Cost: Cheap and fun as recreational sport. Reasonable when played at club level.
Convenience: Easy to organise informal games, very adaptable to numbers.
Sociability: Very good. Game played to

win within rules therefore enjoyable. Teams friendly and welcoming to newcomers.
Difficulty/Skill: Recreationally, minimal skills to hit and catch a ball. Harder for special skills of pitcher and catcher. At social level, no training effect. Competitively, must develop catching, throwing and striking skills as well as sprinting.
Muscles Used: *Pitcher*—shoulder, back, chest, arm muscles. *Catcher*—quads, hamstrings and calves getting up and down. Strengthen hips, shoulder, biceps and wrists for batting.
Wear and Tear: Injuries usually due to someone unfit trying to do too much. Otherwise: *Pitchers*—blisters on throwing hand; elbow strain if pitching more than 3 times per week. *Catchers*—mallet finger due to ball hitting it. Ankle injuries when changing direction quickly when running. But in fact injuries rare.
Time: Game can take whole afternoon or evening. Little fitness benefit considering time spent.
Specific Tips: Practise catching and throwing in spare moments.

Pregnancy: A, B, C—1   Over 50
           A, B—2

Surfing

Riding waves on a special board.
Cost: Recreational surfing is cheap: hire a board or buy secondhand. As you improve specialist or quality boards become expensive. Wetsuits expensive.
Convenience: Long distance travel often needed to find suitable weather and good waves.
Difficulty/Skill: Not easy to start with, but once initial problems overcome and you can get on the board, quite easy to practise; practise to improve. Big gulf between competent recreational surfer and competitor. To start, must have basic confidence in water, swimming ability and good balance.
Sociability: Recreational surfing as part of yachting or windsurfing (boardsailing) or water-skiing club very social. Competitive surfing very individual.
Muscles Used: Arms and shoulders need strength and flexibility in order to paddle out to sea. Ankles, back and particularly calves and quadriceps used to control balance and direction of board.
Wear and Tear: Knees (—eg, torn cartilages in professionals) due to stress from holding position and turning sharply. Cuts or bruises from falls in shallow water, rocks, or on board itself.
Time: Initially, many repeated attempts, but once mastered not forgotten, like cycling.
Specific Tips: Build up arms and shoulders, and ensure flexibility in back and knees. Beware sunburn and wetsuit rub.

Pregnancy: A, B—1

Swimming

Offers all-round fitness for any age or state of health.
Cost: Minimal—bathing suit, cap and goggles, plus entry fee to pool.
Convenience: There are swimming pools in almost every large town in the world. If you live near coast, river or lake, you are lucky!
Difficulty/Skill: Learning to swim is easiest when you are very young and fearless. But even for an adult, swimming is not difficult. Recreational swimming can be as gentle or as hard as you like. Competitive swimming *is* hard, requiring commitment in training—both in the pool and out.
Sociability: Good—especially if you are a member of a club or team. Can take whole family swimming.
Muscles Used: All (see p. 38). Good for toning up stomach and pelvic floor muscles and for working out when you are injured or have a bad back. Excellent for pregnancy. Good heart/lung activity.
Wear and Tear: Nil.
Time: As much as or as little as you wish, unless competitive.
Specific Tips: Wear goggles to protect eyes from chlorine, wear cap to keep hair off face. Remove all jewellery.

Pregnancy: A, B—1   Over 50
        A, B, C, D—2, 3

Table Tennis

Bat and ball game played across low net on table.
Cost: Cheap, though good shoes and bat worth investment.
Convenience: Widely available at low cost in clubs and sports halls and leisure centres. But clubs usually just to practise and play matches, so hard for adult to start unless you buy own table etc.
Sociability: Clubs tend to cater only to competitive, so not as good as may be.
Difficulty/Skill: Enjoyable by all ages with little or no fitness needed. Some hand/eye co-ordination needed, and ability to hit ball.
Muscles Used: In competitions, great agility, power, speed needed. Also reflexes as well as flexibility, and strength in hips, legs, back, arms and wrists.
Wear and Tear: Lower back and shoulder strain, tennis elbow and ankle sprains common among top 5% of players. Due to overuse and heavy top-spin/looped play. No injuries at lower levels.
Time: Little time spent at recreation level means little training effect. To play seriously extra fitness training needed to improve stamina, reflexes and flexibility.
Specific Tips: No problems unique to women. Fully equal chance—not dependent on strength and power. All national events open to both men and women and doubles and mixed doubles popular.

| Pregnancy: A, B, C, D—1 | Over 50 |
| A, B, C—2 | |

Ta'i Chi Chuan

Japanese martial art.
Cost: Reasonable as teaching is on individual or small group basis.
Convenience: Widespread availability of teaching but majority poor standard and unqualified. (For example, only two qualified schools in London. Beware imitations.)
Difficulty/Skill: No pre-requisites at all. Requires commitment to see the course through which is minimum of six months.
Sociability: Like many oriental arts involving mental discipline, concentration is on individual body and mind.
Muscles Used: Very good for fitness and health.
Wear and Tear: External, physical strength not relevant therefore women can work with men on equal terms. Also no injuries—even when used as a martial art.
Time: Minimum one session per week, perhaps more at start. Six months to learn whole pattern of basics, then work with partner.
Specific Tips: Many T'ai Chi recruits are going to it from aerobics, jogging etc, and finding it much more rewarding because of mental element.

| Pregnancy: A, B—1 | Over 50 |

Tennis

Racket and ball sport played over a low net on a court.
Cost: Clothing not expensive, but racket and footwear can be, although worth getting quality as it will help to play, is comfortable and lasts a long time. Public courts cheap. Clubs not dear. Indoor facilities can be more expensive.
Convenience: Plenty of public courts available, but not always good surface. Private clubs common, many now with indoor facilities.
Sociability: Tennis clubs very social and good way to meet others and find someone of similar level. Club sessions geared to intermixing players of different skills, experience and sexes. Many clubs organise social activities.
Difficulty/Skill: Social tennis at lowest level does not require high level fitness but game improves quickly if fitter. General co-ordination required to hit moving ball. Easy game to take up gently. Practice needed to improve. No previous experience required but eye/hand co-ordination important.
Muscles Used: Legs, hips, biceps, triceps, and shoulders. Serving increases flexibility in shoulders. Reaching and bending limbers up

knees, hips, backs of legs. Also strengthens wrists and forearm of racket arm.
Wear and Tear: Elbow, shoulder soreness. Short dashes forward, back, and sideways, and changes of direction put stress on all lower limbs. Aches and pains, especially tennis elbow, often caused by poor technique. Blisters on hand and feet (check grip and fitting of socks and shoes).
Time: As a gentle social game, once a week probably contributes nothing to fitness. Need to play hard, full matches two or three times a week to gain some aerobic and flexibility benefit. To improve further, must also work on stamina (eg, bicycling) and intervals to improve sprint speed.
Specific Tips: Your basic social tennis will improve dramatically as you get fitter, because you'll be able to hit shots the way you are supposed to.

Pregnancy: A, B—1   Over 50

Volleyball

6-a-side team game; ball is propelled over a high central net.
Cost: Clubs, low cost membership. Kit not expensive, though good footwear important.
Convenience: Purely recreational. Growing quickly around the world. Can be played outdoors or indoors, even on the beach.
Difficulty/Skill: Very easy to play casually and informally. Practice and coaching needed to develop expertise. Can start at most clubs without experience.
Sociability: Very good at both recreational and competitive level, and full of enthusiasts.
Muscles Used: Calves, thighs, hamstrings, arms, shoulders and wrists. Everything associated with jumping.
Wear and Tear: Damaged fingers, ankle and knee injuries common to all jumping sports.
Time: Games and training sessions would take at least two 2-hour sessions a week. Playing recreationally and enthusiastically on the beach is energy-consuming.

SPORT AND EXERCISE GUIDE

Specific Tips: The greater suppleness of women, if combined with fitness and acquired skills, make women very good volleyball players.

Pregnancy: A, B, C—1, 2   Over 50

Water Polo

7-a-side team game, like basketball in the water. Goals scored in soccer type goal.
Cost: Low.
Convenience: Most swimming centres also have water polo clubs either part of club or separate club. Still new for women however.
Sociability: As it's new, once you're in a club full of enthusiasts you have common interest.
Difficulty/Skill: One of the most strenuous sports. Takes years to develop the swimming, strength, and ball-handling skills to be a good competitive player.
Muscles Used: All-over strength and flexibility. Powerful swimmer. High body position in water vital, therefore strong legs, abdominals, and back required.
Wear and Tear: Impact injuries—cuts and abrasions from clashes with arms and elbows, common. Overuse problems in the shoulders. As no goggles worn, eye prone to chlorine irritation.
Time: Terrific stamina demands require extensive training in addition to team and skills practice.
Specific Tips: Wear ear pads to prevent damage from elbows etc.

Pregnancy: A—1

Waterskiing

Towed behind boat on skis doing various tricks, jumps and slalom moves.
Cost: Expensive—due hire of boat, skis and wetsuit.
Convenience: Considerable now on lakes, reservoirs, gravel pits and sea.
Difficulty/Skill: For recreational water skiing, no special training needed after basic skills taught and learnt. Competitively, coaching, great stamina, and strength needed.

153

Generally, strength needed in forearms, shoulders, quadriceps, buttocks, and abdomen.
Sociability: As clubs are limited to boardsailing and yachting clubs they are well organised and very social.
Muscles Used: All: legs, arms, shoulders, trunk, and back—especially thighs and shoulders. Flexibility in back improved. Good for toning muscle if ski regularly.
Wear and Tear: Strain from overuse, especially if technique poor. At competition level, torn knee cartileges and ligaments. Recreational, thighs, lower back and aching arms.
Time: Stamina and strength needs building elsewhere—two or three times per week to have training effect. Regular sessions on holiday can be effective.
Specific Tips: If speedskiing, wear helmet to protect from head injuries in fall.

Pregnancy: A—1   Over 50

Weight Training

Programme of gradual muscle strengthening by use of free weights or special machinery and equipment, eg variable resistance apparatus. Not to be confused with weightlifting, which is a competitive sport.
Cost: Weight training should be carried out in a gym under qualified supervision. Fee for membership usually low but if you buy own equipment this can be expensive.
Convenience: Facilities increasingly available at gyms and fitness centres. After you have trained into a supervised programme, can work out at home also.
Difficulty/Skill: No special skill needed; a simple, if repetitive way to get fit and you can work at a level to suit yourself. Weights graded from easy-to-lift at first, more strenuous as you get stronger.
Muscles Used: Specific exercises can work out every muscle in the body, but expert advice needed on correct technique, weight and frequency of lifts. Joints strengthened and become more injury-resistant. Not an aerobic activity, so supplement with swimming or cycling.
Wear and Tear: Under controlled conditions, no injuries should occur. Enthusiasts may risk strains from muscle imbalance or overuse.
Time: Regular workouts—three hourly sessions per week—are needed to register improvement. Should include proper warm up and gradual wind down.
Specific Tips: An essential complement to serious sports competition: can improve muscular strength, endurance, stamina, posture and co-ordination.

Windsurfing

The cheapest form of sailing: a surfboard with a sail on it.
Cost: Medium price as lessons and board hire essential. Once competent, boards quite expensive. Wetsuit needed. Board transportable on roof of car.
Convenience: Now widespread on inland waters, often in conjunction with yacht clubs. Good fun if you live nearby.
Difficulty/Skill: Swimming competence and confidence in water needed, otherwise no aptitude or experience or strengths. Soon learn with a little help and even basic boardsailing is fun. Practice needed to get better and cope with stronger winds.
Sociability: Clubs very social, and excellent places to meet and be coached. Any standard welcome and no experience needed to join. Cameraderie of 'boom' sport, often in conjunction with yacht clubs and water skiing.
Muscles Used: Upper body strength—especially for beginner when tense. Back, arms, and legs—especially forearms and quadriceps. Flexibility in hips, shoulders, legs, and groin.
Wear and Tear: Hand blisters, soreness in lower back, legs, calves and ankles. Board very safe—floats, stops dead as soon as sail hits water so you can hold on or sit on it. Serious injuries rare though ignorance of wind and tides can result in tragedies at sea.
Time: A little experienced guidance plus trial and error will soon enable you to start and stay aboard in gentle wind.

After that, the more you do, the faster you improve. Makes a fun holiday.
Specific Tips: Women have advantages over men as they are lighter. Therefore board is faster and women can often beat men in equal competition.

Pregnancy: A, B—1

Wrestling

Contact sport. Object, to pin opponent to floor. The oldest form of sport in the world.
Cost: As in martial arts. Helps to join and work with a martial art—ie, Judo or Aikido before and while wrestling.
Convenience: Growing, but not widespread either in the UK or US.
Difficulty/Skill: No experience or natural skill required except competitiveness and aggression. Can continue for many years, peak in 40s. Natural gymnastic ability and balance is important as well as courage.
Muscles Used: Every muscle and joint into action either to bring pressure to bear on opponent or to escape. Proper 'Breakfall' must be learnt through martial arts.
Wear and Tear: Cuts, scrapes, and bruises are part for the course. Join injuries, particularly knees, shoulders and lower back. Most injuries come from failure to react quickly or correctly, or to fall correctly.
Time: Considerable, must get to good standard in martial arts first.
Specific Tips: Very good for women as naturally 60% stronger in legs than arms and wrestling demands leg strength. Strategy and technique just as important as strength. Women should only wrestle with women.

Yoga

Indian physical and mental discipline that keeps muscles toned as well as mind clear.
Cost: Cheap. Classes run for groups.
Convenience: Classes widespread, both private and public facilities. Can do anywhere, anytime to suit self after basics mastered.

Sociability: Done in groups, so shared experience but essentially 'individual' activity. All accepted.
Difficulty/Skill: No pre-requisites. Fitness or good shape not required.
Muscles Used: Entire body brought into use in gentle, calculated manner. Breathing aided by control techniques being learnt.
Wear and Tear: None. Controlled, gentle nature of exercise should produce no damage at all. Session should yield relaxation and well being.
Time: Need to commit to introductory sessions to learn basic techniques. After that formal classes can be less regular (although still a good thing). Once a week ideal. As much time as want at home.
Specific Tips: Excellent way of relaxing and coping with stress. Excellent contrast to aerobic activity like jogging and no reason for self-consciousness at start due to inexperience or physique. Can help bring down high blood pressure.

Pregnancy: A, B, C, D— 1, 2   Over 50

WOLVERHAMPTON PUBLIC LIBRARIES

Index

A

abdomen:
    muscles 27, 36, 72, 74, 82, 84, 125, 128
    operations 130-3
    post-operative exercise 131-3
aches and pains 26, 27, 32, 42, 43, 50
    menstrual 62-3
    post-injury 52
    stress 105
achilles tendon, 33, 128
    protector 31
acupressure 115
adrenalin 104, 106
aerobics 41
age 26
    ageing 26, 87, 89
    brittle bones 87
    cycling 38
    training 60, 61
aikido 134
alcohol 97, 108-10
    foetal alcohol syndrome 109
    problem drinking 109
    skin and 116, 118, 119
    sleep and 111
amenorrhoea 63, 75
American Skin Cancer Foundation 117
anaemia 62, 78
anaerobic exercise 41, 60
ankles 128
    sprains 53
    swelling 68
anorexia nervosa 61, 110
anti-perspirant 123
appendicectomy 130
appestat 93, 101
appetite 93

archery 134
armpits 122-3
arms 123, 124-5
arteries 10
arthritis 27, 96, 123
asthma 27
athlete's foot 129

B

baby:
    physical development 16-18
back 123
    low back pain 27
    spondylolysis 60
badminton 135
balance 53
    in pregnancy 73, 75
barefoot 129
    babies 18
    dance 42
baseball 60, 150-1
basketball 135-6
Benoit, Joan 60
bio feedback 115
black toe 129
bladder:
    frequency 65
    menopause 86
    stress incontinence 79
blisters 30, 145
blood:
    glucose level 93, 97, 101
    high blood pressure 26, 68
boardsailing 154
body:
    body-image 81
    care 116-129
    major changes 54-89
    physical development 16-22
    shape 28-29
    structure and injury 51-2
body building 136
bones:
    brittle (osteoporosis) 38, 87
    childhood injury 60
bottom 128
bowling 136-7
bowls 136-7
bra:
    pregnancy 73
    sports 30, 73, 123
breakfast 92
breasts 123
    exercises 126-7
    lumpectomy 133
    mastectomy 133
breathing:
    diaphragmatic 113
    yoga 112
breathlessness 78
British Disabled Waterski Association 14
bulimia nervosa 110

C

Caesarian section 133
caffeine 97
calcium 58, 87, 102-3
calories 90, 92
    and exercise 101
Callen, Kenneth E 33
canoeing 137
Cantu, Dr Robert 12
cap *see* diaphragm
carbohydrate 96, 97
    sources of 102
chewing gum 120
child:
    athletic child abuse 60-1
    effects of smoking on 107
    physical abilities 20
    physical development 16-22
    sport for 21-2
    sports injuries 61
childbirth 73
cholecystectomy 130
cholesterol 93
cigarettes 106
circuit training 137
climbing 138
clothing, *see* sportswear
coil, *see* intra-uterine device
cold:
    and cycling 39
    exposure 50
    skin protection 118
Committee on the Paediatric Aspects of Physical Fitness, Recreation and Sports 21
conception 68
constipation:
    and pregnancy 81
    and premenstrual tension 64
contact lenses 119
contact sports:
    and joints 52
    in pregnancy 84-5
    protection of mouth 120
contraception:
    the Pill 62, 65, 107
    and sport 65
convenience, *see* individual sports
Cooper, Dr Kenneth H 41
Cosgrave, Bill 19
cost, *see* individual sports
cramp 58, 128
cricket 138
cycling 138
    basic exercise plan 38-41, 46-9
    bicycle 38
    during pregnancy 84-5
    osteoporosis and 38, 87
    post-operative 130
    sportswear 30, 39

INDEX

D

dance 139
   basic exercise plan 41-2, 46-9
   clothing 42
   shoes 42
dental care 120
deodorant 123
depression 27, 102, 81
diabetes 27, 101
diaphragm 65
Diem, Prof Lieselote 16
diet, 10, 90-103
   calories 90, 92
   healthy eating 96-7
   and menstruation 58
   see also eating; food; nutrition
dieting:
   during pregnancy 81
Dines, Alison 15
disability:
   and exercise 14-15
   British Disabled Waterski Association 14
disc, slipped 27
discipline 43
diving 139-40
   scuba 148
drugs:
   for dysmenorrhoea 63
   during pregnancy 45
dysmenorrhoea 62-3

E

ears 117, 120
   plugs 120
East Germany 12
eating:
   breakfast 92
   compulsive 110
   and exercise 101
   exercise after 128
   problems 104
   see also diet; food; nutrition
ectomorph 29
Einon, Dorothy: 'Creative Play' 22
elbows 122
   golfer's elbow 140
   tennis elbow 123
endomorph 29
endorphins 27, 35
energy 24, 92
environment 50
epilepsy 26
equipment:
   and injury 50
exercise 8
   appetite and 93
   basic plan 42-9
   benefits 9
   depression and 27
   disabled and 14-5
   during pregnancy 66-85
   eating 101, 110
   heart and 8, 10
   in infancy 19-20
   menopause and 86
   menstruation and 61-4
   mentally handicapped 15
   over 50s 87-9
   post-operative 130-3
   post-natal 81-3
   premenstrual tension and 64
   puberty and 54-61
   smoking and 26, 108
   starting 24-49
   stress and 106
exercise bicycle 39, 144
eyebrows 119
eyes 119
   contact lenses 119
   goggles 119
   infections 120
   make-up 120
   problems 119-20
eyesight 120

F

face 118-21
fat cells 58
fatigue 50
   post-natal 81
   pregnancy 73, 75
fats 96, 97
   cutting down 98
   sources 102
feet 128-9
   athlete's foot 129
   baby's 18
   barefoot 129
   massage 115
   shoes 30, 31
fellrunning 146
fencing 140
fibre 58, 81, 96
   sources 102
fingers 123
fitness 8
   and housewives 12
   pregnancy 68
   pulse test 25
fluid retention 64
foetal alcohol syndrome 109
food:
   additives 96
   constituents of 90
   cooking, buying and eating 94, 99
   daily intake 102-3
   eating problems 110
   richest sources 102-3
   see also diet; eating; nutrition
foot, *see* feet
footwear 30, 31
   barefoot 18, 42, 129
Francis, Dr Peter R 129
fungal infection 129

G

gall bladder 130
   cholecystectomy 130
games:
   infancy 19, 22
   organised 22
girls and sport 21-2
glasses, dark 119
gloves 123
goggles 119
   swimming 35, 119
golf 140
   golfer's elbow 140
groin 128
growth:
   childhood 21
   infancy 16
Guillebaud, Dr John 107
gumshield 120
Guttmann, Prof Ludwig 14
gymnastics 140-1
   'Tumble Tots' 19

H

hair 118
handball 141
hands 123
   lefthandedness 18
Hawley, Anne: 'Swim, Baby, Swim' 17
head 118
Health Education Council 58
hearing 120
heart:
   disease 12, 26, 93, 107
   and exercise 8, 10
   fitness test 25
   pulse rate 10
heel:
   achilles tendon 33, 128
   Sever's disease 60
hiking 32
hips 44-5, 128
hockey 141-2
housewives 12
hunger 93
hypoglycaemia 101
   and premenstrual tension 64
hysterectomy 131

I

I.C.E. (ice – compression – elevation) 52
ice hockey 142
ice skating 142
illness 50
incontinence, stress 79

157

INDEX

infancy:
    exercise and play 19
    feet 5
    growth 16
    infant deaths 38, 107
    lefthandedness 18
    physical development 18
    swimming 16-7
injury:
    acute 52-3
    chronic 53
    massage 114
    pregnancy and 75
    prevention 50
    puberty 60-1
    resuming exercise 53
    through overuse 50
interval training 142-3
intra-uterine device (IUD) 65
iron 58, 102-3
Irvine, Marion 89

J

'jock itch' 128
jogging 143-4
    basic exercise plan 32-5, 46-9
    sportswear 30, 33
    trails 33
joints:
    arthritis 27, 96, 123
    child 61
    loose 51-2
judo 143

K

Kabisch, Dr 12
karate 145
kayaking 137
knees 128
    knock-knees 51
Koch, Dr 17
Kristiansen, Ingrid 75
kung fu 145

L

lacrosse 143-4
lefthandedness 18
legs 128
    bow-legs 51
leotard 42
'Let's Play to Grow' 15
liberation through sport 13
lips 120
lumpectomy 133

M

machines, exercise 144
make-up 118, 120
marathon running 144-5
Margaret Morris Movement 41-2

martial arts 145
    and joints
massage 114
mastectomy 126, 132-3
Masters, Dr William: 'Human Sexual Response' 63
medau 145
medicine, preventive 12
meditation 115
menarche 56
men, women compared with 12, 33, 60
menopause 86-7
    and heart disease 93
menstruation 61-3
    amenorrhoea 63, 75
    calendar 64
    dysmenorrhoea 62
    exercise and 63
    menarche 56-7
    physiological effects 62
    premenstrual tension 64
mental handicap 15
mesomorph 29
metabolism 101
milk 58, 98
    skimmed 94, 98
minerals, see vitamins and minerals
'Mini-Pill' 65
miscarriage 78
    and smoking 107
mobility, post-injury 53
Morris, Prof Jeremy 12
Morris, Margaret 41-2
mother and baby classes 17
motor skills 19, 21
mountaineering, see climbing
Moutawakel, Nawal El 13
mouth 120
    mouthguard 120
    mouthwash 120
multi-gym 144
muscles:
    face 119, 121
    fast and slow twitch fibre 28
    injury 52-3, 63
    muscle-bound 58, 60
    pelvic floor 79, 80, 129
    relaxation 113
    toning 44-5, 69-74, 79, 82-3, 122, 124-5, 126-7, 129-31, 132

N

nails 123
neck 120, 122
netball 145-6
nicotine 106
nipples 117
nose 117, 120
nutrition 90-103
    see also diet; eating; food

O

oestrogen 54, 57, 58
    and heart disease 93, 107
operations, abdominal 130
orienteering 35, 146
orthotics 31
Osgood-Schlatter's disease 60
osteoporosis 87
over weight 26
ovulation 64

P

pacing yourself 32
Paffenbarger, Dr Ralph 12
pain, see aches and pains
parcours 146
parents 19
    as coaches 22
patience 43
pattering 43
pelvic floor:
    exercises 72, 79, 129
    muscles 80
period, see menstruation
physical development:
    childhood 20-1
    infancy 16-18
    puberty 54
pill, contraceptive 62, 65
    and smoking 107
play 19-22
play pens 19
post-natal depression 81
post-natal exercises 82-83
posture 27, 41, 115, 124, 125
potatoes 96
pregnancy 66-85
    alcohol and 68, 109
    exercise during 73-81
    fears 75-8
    injury during 75
    posture 74
    preparation for 68
    smoking 107
    sportswear 73
    training effect of 81
    weight gain 78-80
premenstrual tension 64
    and alcohol
progesterone 78
pronation 31
protective equipment 50
proteins 96, 97
    sources 102
psychology in puberty 61
puberty 54-61
pulse rate 10
    as fitness guide 25
    in pregnancy 73
pulses 96

INDEX

R

rambling 32
Read, Dr Malcolm 61
reflexes:
    in cycling 39
    in infancy 16
reflexology 115
relaxation 111-5
    during pregnancy 67, 73, 81
Richards, Gordon 43
riding 146
    and pregnancy 75
rock climbing 138
rollerskating 147
rope jumping 150
rowing 147
    machine 144
rugby 148
running 143
    basic exercise plan 32-5, 46-9
    fell 146
    marathon 144
    old age 87, 89
    on roads 33
    on sand 33
    runner's high 35
    runner's knee 128
    sportswear 30, 33
    from stress 104

S

sailing 148
salt 64, 96, 97
sanitary wear 57-8
schools 12
scuba diving 148-9
Seddington, Ken 60
Sever's disease 60
sex 63
sexual stereotyping 21
sheath 65
shiatsu 115
shin 60
shoes 30, 31
shoulders 120-2
Shriver, Eunice Kennedy 15
skiing:
    alpine 149
    cross-country 85, 149-50
    pregnancy and 75, 85
skin:
    care of 116-8
    cleansing 118-9
    moisture 116
    sun 116-7
skipping 150
sleep 111
    and premenstrual tension 64
slipped disc 21
smoking 26, 106-8
    skin and 117
soccer 150
sociability: *see* individual sports
Socialism and sport 12
softball 150-1
spare tyre 125
spermicide 65
spondylolysis 60
sport:
    child 21, 22
    woman 12-12
    see also individual sports
sportswear 30
    cycling 30, 39
    dance 30, 42
    during pregnancy 73
    running 30, 33
    shoes 30, 31
    swimming 35
    walking 30, 32
starch 96
sterilisation 131
stitch 124
stomach, *see* abdomen
strength:
    increasing 52, 154
    regaining 53
stress 104-6
    and amenorrhoea 63
    and premenstrual tension 64
    and skin 118
stress incontinence 79
stretching 44-5
    for muscle injury 53
    warming up 44-5, 50
stride jumps 79
Stuart, Nik 19
sugar 96
    cutting down 98
sunlight 116-8, 119
    protection 117
sunbed 119
sunglasses 119
supination 31
surfing 151-2
surgery 130-3
sweating 72, 73
swimming 151
    baby 16-17
    basic exercise plan 35-8, 46-9
    cap 35
    cramp 128
    earplugs 120
    goggles 35
    hair care 118
    pool exercises 36-7
    post-operative 130
    pregnancy 73, 74, 75, 78
    strokes 38
    swimsuit 35

T

table tennis 152
tae kan do 145
ta'i chi chuan 152
talk test 33, 41
tampons 58
targets 32
technique 50
teeth 120
    toothguard 120
tennis 152-3
    tennis elbow 123
thighs 128
thrush 128
tiredness, *see* fatigue
toes 129
toothguard 120
tracksuit 30
training:
    injury 50
    puberty 60
'Tumble Tots' 19
tummy, *see* abdomen

U/V

unfit 12, 24
varicose veins 133
Vegans 99
verrucas 129
vitamins and minerals 99-100
    and premenstrual tension 64
    sources 102
    vitamin deficiency 107, 108
volleyball 153

W/Y

walking:
    basic exercise plan 32
    post-operative 130, 133
    pregnancy 73, 85
    sportswear 30, 32
warming up 33
water polo 153
waterskiing 153-4
wear and tear, *see* individual
    sports
weather 50
weight:
    amenorrhoea 63
    ideal 24, 28
    overweight 26
    pregnancy 78-9
    puberty 58-9
    smoking and 108
weights 124-5
weight training 154
Wilmore, Dr J H 58
windsurfing 154
wobble board 53
women:
    and fitness 9
    compared to men 12, 33, 60
wrestling 155
wrists 123
yoga 122, 156
yoghurt 94, 128

Acknowledgements

Breslich & Foss would like to thank the following for their help and co-operation:
Jan and Graham Smith and the Optimum Health Club, St Ives, Cambridgeshire, Debbie Rudd of Arena UK, Mike Cowper of Mike Cowper Photography, Jan Callini, Eileen Dessaso, Emma Davis, Jane Ewing, Judy Ewing, Michaela Haggarty, Tania Hester, Natalie Lill, Vicky Lill, Anne Nichols, and Anita O'Carroll. Also, Ian Coussins at the St Ivo Outdoor Complex, and Mike Hunt, Recreation Supervisor at the St Ivo Recreation Centre, St Ives, Cambridgeshire.

The publisher also wishes to thank the following for permission to quote from copyright material:
Anne Hawley *Swim, Baby, Swim*, Pelham Books, 1984
Dorothy Einon *Creative Play*, Duncan Petersen Publishing Ltd, 1985

Picture Credits

P 13   Organisers of the London Marathon.

P 14   British Disabled Water Ski Association.

P 17   Ian Hickley-Smith.

P 19   Tumble Tots.

P 55, 88   The Embassy of the Federal Republic of Germany, London.

While information contained in this book is in accordance with reputable medical opinion, the authors and the publisher are not responsible for any adverse consequences resulting from the interpretation, use or misuse of any of the suggestions, recommendations, sports or exercises mentioned in this book.